The Complete Book of
Water Therapy

Keats Titles of Related Interest

THE COMPLETE BOOK OF WATER THERAPY

Dian Dincin Buchman

Illustrations by Blanche Fried

Keats Publishing, Inc. ⚹ New Canaan, Connecticut

The Complete Book of Water Therapy is not intended as medical advice. Its intent is solely informational and educational. Please consult a health professional should the need for one be indicated.

THE COMPLETE BOOK OF WATER THERAPY

Copyright © 1994 by Dian Dincin Buchman

All Rights Reserved

An earlier edition of this book was published in 1979 by E. P. Dutton; this edition incorporates a new chapter and substantial updating and revision.

No part of this book may be reproduced in any form without the written consent of the publisher.

Library of Congress Cataloging-in-Publication Data

Buchman, Dian Dincin.
    The complete book of water therapy / Dian Dincin Buchman :
  illustrations by Blanche Fried.—[Rev. and updated]
      p.   cm.
  Includes index.
   ISBN 0-87983-613-X : $11.95
   1. Hydrotherapy.   I. Title.
RM811.B78   1994
615.8'53—dc20   93-47004
                                           CIP

Printed in the United States of America

Published by Keats Publishing, Inc.
27 Pine Street (Box 876)
New Canaan, Connecticut 06840-0876

This book is dedicated to
CAITLIN DINCIN BUCHMAN

Contents

Appendixes

Foreword

I grew up in a family that truly enjoyed doing most things naturally. We used water—especially cold water—as our *primary* health aid, and many other water treatments for the prevention and remedy of minor health problems. In our daily arsenal we used hot and cold compresses, showers, short "dunks," long baths, as well as dozens of other water techniques, and we always knew how to quickly overcome fatigue, sore throat, and colds. In fact, with our knowledge of water, herbs, and exercise we rarely needed "heavy" doctoring. We drowned incipient colds with determined water drinking, detoxifying baths, and perspiration-inducing herbal teas. We also used many kinds of off-the-shelf home products, as well as everyday foods, our garden flowers, and herbs in various forms, in our home ministrations. Because we had constant success with these treatments, we never hesitated to use them for emergency first aid for cuts, bumps, sprains, burns, delayed or protracted menstrual periods, or the ordinary health problems that occur daily.

A Return to Old Health Values

During my childhood all these things had seemed so effortless that as I grew up I was bewildered to discover that other people used complicated medicines to get the same effects that we achieved with only water. I was stunned when I discovered that my neighbors and friends requested antibiotics for even the most minor ailment.

To my present chagrin, at one point in my late teens and early twenties, I just didn't want to feel—or be—different from all these other people, and I joined them. It wasn't until I became *less* energetic, and my husband and child seemed to be ill more often, that I decided to retrieve all my inherited knowledge of natural healing, and also to investigate other forms of nondrug health approaches. My family's remarkable range of water therapies proved to be one of the exciting answers in my quest for knowledge.

My Health Roots

In *her* girlhood, my maternal grandmother had a short, but extraordinary, contact with Rumanian gypsies. She taught me many native and gypsy remedies that used plants and household foods. But it was the Dincins, my father's family, who taught us water therapy concepts. Many of my father's uncles and other relatives were "old-fashioned" physicians who believed in the body's natural ability to heal itself when properly stimulated. They were, and are, a very adventurous group. One had traveled to Worishaven, Bavaria, to observe how the great nineteenth century master Sebastian Kneipp conducted his "water cure" therapies. He also studied with Dr. Wilhelm Winternitz, the Austrian scientist who researched the direct and indirect nerve reactions from water. This great uncle then joined with other pioneers and investigated the action of various states of water on the human body and, together with other forward-thinking physicians and lay healers, utilized water within their private and hospital practice.

Uncle Doc and Cold Water

My father's uncle, Dr. Herman Dincin, worked with all the early, great exponents of American hydrotherapy. Among them was the outstanding Dr. Simon Baruch, the physician who actually brought hydrotherapy to America. At first this system was received indifferently, but later it was used by some of the great internists, including Sir William Osler.

Several of these clinically minded physician-hydrotherapists wrote papers or books on their experiences. Among those I and my father's family are deeply indebted to include Dr. William Dieffenbach, a Professor of Bacteriology at New York Medical College and Hospital for Women, and later a Professor of Hydrotherapy at Flower Hospital; the great health reformer, Dr. J. H. Kellogg, who advised lay people on the "Uses of Water in Health and Disease"; various physicians for religious groups that stressed nondrug medicine, among them Dr. George Knapp Abbott, Dean of Faculty, Professor of Physiology, and Superintendent of the Loma Linda Hospital in California; and Dr. R. Lincoln Graham, the inventor of the graham cracker, who also wrote "Water in Disease and in Health," and who achieved astonishing cures with water.

Although Uncle Herman was first a family doctor and then an endocrinologist, his secret passion was plain old water therapy. Our family had always used the simple double throat compress (a cold water compress followed by a wool bandage to keep out air), and various other cold water packs and compresses. Uncle Herman taught me about cold water foot splashes and cold water treading to increase disease resistance, and the value of the circulation-inducing and inexpensive pickup: the coarse salt rubdown before a bath. He explained to me how and why these and innumerable other water therapy techniques worked on the body.

This book is a product of all I have learned from my family, plus the knowledge I have gained from over twenty years of investigating the principles and dynamics of water as therapy. As a Ph.D. in health science, with a special area of concentration in the chemical properties of water and water's physiological action on the body, I have had the opportunity to explore in depth how water affects the human body and, especially, how it can be used to promote good health. This knowledge, plus the experience I have gained from teaching and lecturing on water therapy and other health-related subjects for several years, is all reflected in this volume.

This book also includes much information that I have acquired over the years talking with numerous physicians, especially sports physicians, orthopedists, neurosurgeons; chiropracters, osteopaths, physiotherapists, rehabilitation experts, head athletic trainers, and hundreds of other sports participants and lay people who use water in special ways to control illness and to maintain good health.

Among the many specialists to whom I am indebted in this search are: Olympic athlete Bruce Jenner; sports physicians Dr. Vincent Di Stephano, team physician for the Philadelphia Eagles, and Dr. Alexander Kalenak, team orthopedic surgeon at Pennsylvania State University; Dr. Isao Hirata, Jr., Director, Student Health Service, University of South Carolina, and former Yale athletic surgeon and team physician for varsity football; the neurosurgeon, Dr. Arthur Winter; Dr. C. Jack Lutt, Assistant Director of Student Services of California State University, Hayward; rehabilitation specialists Jack M. Hofkosh, Director of Physical Therapy, New York University Medical Center, Institute of Rehabilitation Medicine, Miss Judith Kurtz, Administrator, Department of Rehabilitation, The Hospital for Special Surgery, and Dr. John Hanks, rehabilitation consultant, Denver Broncos, Denver Nuggets; athletic trainers William E. "Pinky" Newell, Head Athletic Trainer, Purdue University, and Mel Blickenstaff, Head Athletic Trainer, Purdue University; Dick Hoover, Suburban Physical Therapy Services, Des Plaines, Illinois; Sayers "Bud" Miller, Athletic Coordinator, Pennsylvania State University; Robert Behnke, Illinois State University, Normal, Illinois; Kenneth Knight, State University College at Brockfort; Gary Delforge, University of Arizona.

Anyone can learn to use water as therapy—for pleasure and to provide better health and more energy.

You will never regret learning the water therapy concepts. Because they are so easy to do, and can be put into effect the minute you start to feel ill, they will make your life less complicated, and ultimately give you more and better *control* of your health.

Dian Dincin Buchman, Ph.D.
New York City
April 1979

Foreword
to the 1994 Edition

Water therapy is a system of natural healing. It uses the body's need for water, and its *physiological responses* to water, to *prevent, correct and treat* a broad range of health and injury problems. These methods, also known as hydrotherapy, were developed in Europe over a century ago, and make up what is one of the least expensive and most versatile and dependable healing systems ever devised.

Water therapy uses stimulation with water to produce subtle changes in energy. All nondrug healing methods, from massage to naturopathy to acupuncture to chiropractic to homeopathy, share some form of energy change. All work to transform static states (illness), into active states (recovery and health).

Water therapy is effective because of body physiology. Not only does the body need water to dissolve, transport and, finally, absorb nutrients; water also extracts and discards waste materials through internal organs, *and through the skin*. Many, but not all, of the remarkable results from water therapy occur through the skin.

The skin is not just the human envelope, it is an extensive, completely accessible organ, the largest organ in the body. One of the functions of the skin is to maintain the body's stable temperature, which is why the skin is particularly sensitive to changes in temperature. Any water application which changes the skin temperature produces an *action*. This in turn causes a *reaction*. This action/reaction generates a third force which initiates self-healing. The dynamics of healing start with small actions. Ovid's axiom is true: "Add a little to a little and there will be a great heap."

Hot, warm, cold water, ice and steam act differently under different circumstances and each is perceived by the skin and thus the internal body as a different product. Also, water has a different result when applied on cloths as compresses or applied with herbs as in poultices. Water can cleanse, can detoxify, and can reduce pain.

Water therapy includes hundreds of remedies, among them several excellent fever treatments, all of which illustrate different solutions (different actions and reactions) to the same problem. 1. Drinking cool water slowly and effectively reduces fever from within the body. 2. Bathing a feverish person in cool, even cold water, immediately reduces fever. 3. Rubbing a feverish person with a cold-friction washcloth-massage reduces the fever by encouraging fresh patterns of circulation. 4. A detoxifying bath utilizes the capacity of the skin to relinquish toxins.

Water therapy remedies work in a variety of ways. The use of a mustard plaster to cure bronchitis is an excellent example of the many effects you can find in water therapy. Teaspoons of powdered mustard, flour and tepid water are placed into a clean cloth, which is folded like an envelope and applied to the chest. This is the *action*. The action works because mustard seed powder is a rubefacient, an irritant that brings blood to the surface of the skin. As the body dispatches blood to the skin's surface through small arterial branches near the capillaries, the freshly circulating blood breaks up the congestion in the chest *from within* the body. This is the *reaction*. Even the harsh internal dry or moist bronchial "rattles" called rales, are no match for this vigorous treatment. Another water therapy for a milder cough is the sipping of plain drinking water, or hot water (like hot lemonade and honey) to expedite the dispersal of phlegm.

Still another interesting example is the cold *double* compress. This technique demonstrates the range and potential of water therapy. In this cold treatment, which eventually deploys heat into the area, the circulating blood breaks up stasis and triggers a recovery. I will describe the use of a cold double compress for a sore throat, but the technique can be used on other parts of the body:

A cold wet cloth, folded in three parts so that it has layers, is fastened closely to the throat, it is then completely covered with a wool scarf. The skin immediately responds to the cold. To equalize its internal temperature the body sends blood to the area. Since the cold compress is encased and *surrounded by the wool scarf,* the internal heat is *trapped* in the area. The healing sorcery begins. Within minutes the blood that starts the healing process from within also warms up the cold compress.

Water has so many other capabilities. *Steam* can open a clogged sinus, or help to extract pollutants and toxins. Solid water—*ice*—can help stop bleeding after injury. Ice prevents further bleeding and circumvents the formation of localized collections of blood called a hematoma.

Ice can also help stop a muscle spasm or an outbreak of herpes or fever blister.

The early practitioners of water therapy thought of cold water as *alive water,* and hot water as "dead." It is true that in water therapy one can get more healing and long-range results with cold water. In fact, one of the great secrets of this form of natural preventive medicine is cold water. It energizes, invigorates, and fortifies the body. One simple yet remarkable example is the use of a daily *cold water* ankle splash to increase resistance to disease.

Cold water works in this way. Cold water applications force the blood vessels to constrict, requiring the blood to travel into another part of the body. At the same time the brain cells, alert to the new unwanted coldness, quickly send fresh blood from the liver to the part of the body receiving the "cold treatment." Within seconds the body is fortified with invigorating, freshly circulating blood.

Cold water treatments afford a great immune system boost by preparing the body for energetic wellness. However, not everyone can use cold water, even in minute amounts. Even in natural healing, *Dios fortiobus adesse,* the gods assist the stronger. Delicate, sickly or frail adults or children will do better with the milder forms of water therapy such as the gentle cold friction rub. In any case, whenever there is a doubt about a treatment, one can never go wrong by using quick alternate hot and cold applications. The alternations produce two mild actions and two equal and opposite reactions which the ailing body utilizes to its best advantage.

This new edition of *Water Therapy* is a result of countless, persistent calls and letters from all over the country from people resolved to track down copies of the original out-of-print publication. I thank these tenacious physicians, massage therapists, body workers, chiropractors, naturopaths and thoughtful people looking for safe holistic answers to good health.

This book re-emerges at an important time. More and more people are seeking reliable self-care approaches to health. At the same time health costs have skyrocketed. We need to have many common-sense preventive methods of healing. I hope this book will help the reader avoid some of the daily health pitfalls that can grow into major health problems. The new edition has an additional chapter with new information on using water therapy for babies, clay and water healing, a new approach to migraine, the relation of water intake to blood pressure, a formula and self test for water intake, the connection between exercise and thirst, appropriate water intake in cold and hot weather exercising, how aging confounds awareness of thirst, dry mouth aids, and a water and homeopathic tip to control dental surgery pain. I also include recent research on adding water to orange juice concentrates, controlling lead pipe leaching into drinking water, and other material.

Dian Dincin Buchman, Ph.D.
New York City, 1994

Acknowledgments

Every investigation has a hidden cadre of generous advisors and aides. I want to thank Vera Stecher, Ph.D., Jean Mundy, Ph.D., Mary Sheerin, Ph.D., and Mary Anne Newman, Ph.D. who helped to focus my studies in hydrotherapy. Caitlin Dincin Buchman, Beatrice Trum Hunter and Ann Reit also helped me.

I want to acknowledge my gratitude for the excellent facilities at the New York Academy of Medicine Library, and the help of Constance Carter of the Library of Congress.

PART I

Water Is

To strengthen the body: pure water to drink,
cold baths, a hair mattress to sleep,
cool air to breathe, and dry food.
—A SCOTTISH SAYING

((1))

Why We Use Water for Therapy

Water Is Holistic Medicine

Water is a natural medicine that benefits the entire body. It can be used in a variety of versatile, no-side-effect ways to help control and cure acute conditions—everything from diarrhea to a cold to migraine headaches—as well as chronic bad health. It can also be used as a disease deterrent, and superior health *safeguard.* The vast number of techniques and therapeutic uses which involve water are collectively known as water therapy, or hydrotherapy. Water therapy, in turn, is a part of a general approach to good health known as *holistic* medicine.

Holistic medicine has several elements: a three-part approach to total health that stresses the interaction of the mind, body, and nutrition; a desire to always investigate the general *cause,* as well as the specific symptom, affecting the body; a need to take responsibility for your own health; a sense of partnership with a caring health practitioner.

In holistic, nondrug medicine, one of the important aims is to overcome sudden or chronic *energy blocks,* and to restore the normal flow of internal energy to the affected part, or to the entire body. Water therapy is a remarkable reenergizer, and can be used in first aid as well as many other everyday problems. In restoring the energy flow, water therapy helps the body to heal itself, and prevents many other health problems from occurring. It is therefore in the first line of health defense, and should be considered an important tool in self-care, and self-*caring* medicine.

A Daily Routine

Water can and should be part of your daily health routine. When you take a warm bath to relax or a short cold shower to stimulate your tired body, you are unconsciously using the techniques of water therapy. I start each day with two personal therapies: I drink two glasses of *cold* water about an hour before breakfast, and I march for a few minutes in a shallow *cold* foot bath. The drinking overcomes an inherited tendency for sluggish peristalsis and the cold water treading boosts my energy and is a long-range body strengthener.

As Simple as Drinking a Glass of Water

Every person who has ever lived on earth has used water for survival, for without drinking water we would die. But because we normally drink water only to quench our thirst, and as a solvent for our foods, we tend to ignore its manifold health benefits and the fact that water is needed internally by every functioning cell and organ.

I've discovered that just drinking a lot of plain, cold water will help to revitalize me during sluggish periods. Physicians and chiropractors often find that weak muscle response, particularly if *all* the muscles are responding in the same way, may be due to minor dehydration. One glass of drinking water sometimes overcomes this strange, total body weakness. Drinking water also can help reduce a high fever, stimulates one organ to interact with another, and cleanses internally by eliminating unwanted material from the system.

Why Water?

What makes treatment with water so unique is that it is always as available as the nearest running water. Moreover, water therapy is *painless,* and hundreds of different health problems can be treated immediately, naturally, and at little or no cost. Water therapy can stop a cold before it starts, help overcome a sore throat, generate energy, relieve pain, vanquish nervousness, help induce sleep, awaken a fogged brain, reestablish internal good health, and even help us to feel sexier; in short, it can restore and tone the body.

What is exceptional about water therapy is that it works with each person's own nature. Water therapy acts in a positive way, and never destroys valuable internal flora, nor does it deplete the energy of internal organs. Water therapy *creates* circulation and overcomes sluggishness; it also unblocks an energy barrier so that the body can function in a freer and normal fashion. By acting to *detoxify*—that is to rid the body of any accumulated poisons or toxins that may be the start of disease, or linger after a disease—water therapy increases our body's natural defense mechanisms.

Dr. William Kellogg, an early twentieth-century advocate of natural foods and natural healing, noted that in perfect health each part of the body receives its due share of blood. Water can equalize the circulation of the blood, control and equalize temperature, relieve pain, stimulate a sluggish or inactive organ, remove foreign or toxic material from the system, and stimulate or soothe the entire nervous system.

Another reason for using the techniques of water therapy is related to the behavior of bacteria in the body. Scientists have discovered that genetic material can jump from one bacterium to another, making them far stronger and more virulent than prior generations of similar bacteria. Dr. Stanley Falkow, of the University of Washington, calls these "jumping genes," and it is his gloomy prediction that more and more bacteria will leap into a new stage. This has happened to *Haemophilus influenzae,* the causative pathogen in some cases of bronchitis, meningitis, pneumonia, and sinusitis. Penicillin used to be able to destroy this bacterium, but now doctors are dismayed to find many patients no longer respond to penicillin treatment.

Scientists have also discovered the alarming fact that other bacteria have become antibiotic-resistant, the way many insects achieved DDT-resistance. More and more virulent strains of certain deadly bacteria are emerging, for example the recent "Legionnaires' Disease," which is now turning up in all parts of the country and which has been classified as an unknown strain of pneumonia. Another example is a new form of typhoid now unresponsive to the antibiotic chloramphenicol. In Mexico, a recent epidemic decimated 14,000 patients before physicians could successfully switch to another antibiotic, in this case, ampicillin.

There is no doubt that antibiotics are successful, but there is also no doubt that the persistent use of antibiotics poses its own dangers. In the natural evolutionary process, any organism will develop successful mutations which are increasingly resistant to the medicines that previously combated them. In the widely hailed British documentary, *The Overworked Miracle,* an American scientist, Dr. Sidney Ross, Chief of Microbiology at the Children's Hospital in Washington, D.C., forecast that this overuse of antibiotics all over the world has created new, and more, deadly diseases. In Dr. Ross's words: "I think we will be looking back fifty years hence, at this as being somewhat of a golden era . . . we may be reverting back to the Middle Ages, as far as antibiotic therapy goes!"

If Dr. Ross's statement is true, and we will have increasing trouble controlling many lethal diseases that are now under control, it will be necessary to reacquire all the forgotten wisdom of nondrug healing. Water therapy—as a serious and effective alternative to toxic drug medicine—is an excellent place to start.

Water for Relaxation

I do not discount the possibility that water therapy is partially effective because it is so enjoyable. Some scientists say we feel better in water because the sea is our true ancestral home. Others liken the feeling of relaxation in water to the memory of the amniotic fluid we were suspended in before birth.

Of the many different water therapies, none is more rewarding than the bath for fun and relaxation. What parent can forget the look of pleasure and security on his newborn infant's face when the LeBoyer warm bath technique is used immediately after birth? Dr. LeBoyer insists that if his postnatal system of quiet, low light, and warm bath were universally practiced, most of us would grow up happier.

Rich or poor, illiterate or scholar, most of us have an inborn instinct about the use of water and stress. An eight-year-old, a battered child, recently confided to a friend of mine that he often took warm baths to relax himself. Once, feeling bereft because his mother had shaved his head as a punishment, he sat in a warm bath for four hours to overcome his seething anger and abject helplessness. He somehow knew instinctually that there was sedation and comfort in that warm bath, just as others instinctively know there is stimulus in a short cold shower. While our feelings about water are to a great extent learned, they may also be part of our collective unconscious, for even the most primitive people used water in a variety of healing ways.

How Water Works in Your Body

Water therapy techniques may be likened to the complex activities in a control tower of a busy airport where takeoffs and landings are a part of a total system whose components must all work together. Some planes land in a center runway. Some are directed to peripheral outlying runways, and still others circle the field, or in bad weather are diverted to other airports. Water can be used in a similar way. It can work directly on the whole body, or it can act on one area to create depletion or congestion.

An example of a direct application of water occurs when you immerse your body in a bath. In this case, the water causes the entire body to feel tonified or sedated. An example of an indirect application of water is the use of a hot foot bath, or of a cold, double wet stocking, to decongest the head or chest during a cold. Another example of an indirect application is the use of a shoulder shower, or an ice bag placed between the thighs, to reduce pelvic congestion.

Learning the many techniques of water therapy is somewhat like studying the superimposed illustrations of the human body that can be found in the *World Book Encyclopedia.* You can view one segment, several superimposed segments, or the total picture, as each celluloid overlay details the circulatory system, the lymphatic system, the endocrine glands, the digestive system, and so on, until the final picture shows the body as we know it.

Water therapy *looks* simple and it is often simple to do, but most of its action is invisible. Water can work in either a simple and direct, or a complex and indirect fashion, and its special therapeutic ability can be employed in its liquid, gas, or solid state.

One of the reasons water is so effective in natural healing is that it stimulates the body by producing an *action* which in turn produces a *reaction.* An example of this is the effect of ice after an injury. The numbing effect of the ice—the action—not only acts as anesthetic and thus reduces pain, but also reduces fluid movement and build-up—the reaction—and this controls bleeding.

The Reflex Arcs

In 1880, Dr. William Winternitz of Austria discovered the startling fact that water acts on the nerve points of the skin. The skin then delivers messages directly to a nearby organ, or *indirectly* through reflex "arcs."

These arcs connect the skin to muscles, glands, and organs. When water—either hot or cold—is applied to the skin, the reflex arcs stimulate nerve impulses that in turn travel to other parts of the body. This action is similar to the transfer of electricity that occurs when a light switch is turned on, or to the effect on a nerve when acupuncture is applied.

Forms of Water

Because water is such a common substance, we tend to take it for granted, never realizing the great variety of its physical and chemical forms that are as easily available to us as the flick of a faucet, making ice cubes, or boiling water in a pot.

Each of these distinctive physical forms of water—ice, water, and steam—must be used differently, for each has its own specific function in healing and in maintaining good health. Indeed, water's therapeutic action is so complex and varied that if water didn't exist, and someone were to invent it today, its inventor would become the most respected and renowned scientist on earth!

Depending on its form (liquid, solid, gas), temperature (cold, hot, ice, neutral), and pressure (light to jet), water will have a specific physical and chemical reaction in, and on, the body.

Cold Water

Cold water acts in several different ways. For example, a short cold-water application acts as a tonic, while an extended cold-water application acts as a depressant.

Basically, however, cold water is *restorative, reenergizing,* and helps *build resistance* to disease. Cold water can help reduce even the highest fever, relieve thirst, act as a stimulant, diuretic, and anesthetic, relieve pain, reduce constipation, and aid the elimination of toxins from the body.

Cold water is the surprising and needed ingredient in a series of excellent *heating* compresses (cold double compress, and various cold double body packs). Unlike hot compresses, which get colder, cold compresses, when trapped by an outer layer of flannel or wool (or even plastic for that matter), become *hot* from heat marshaled from *within* the body.

Ice and Ice Water

Ice, or ice water, is very helpful in reducing the pain of minor burns. Ice massage, or wrapped ice, is the preferred treatment for injuries, as the cold helps to control the bleeding and reduce subsequent swelling. This is the best of all treatments for all sorts of athletic injuries. Ice is an excellent anesthetic.

Warm (Neutral) Water

Warm water is sedating, relaxes the body, and when necessary it is an effective emetic.

Hot Water

Hot water (as well as cold) can be used internally and externally.

In an injury, heat increases blood flow, and will act to increase any inflammation; as a result, hot water must be avoided in treating injuries. However, heat can sedate, quiet, and soothe the body under many other conditions. A short hot-water application depresses and depletes body and muscle tone, making the body feel more relaxed. And while a long hot-water application both excites and depresses the body, the total effect is one of complete relaxation.

Some of the most important therapeutic uses of hot water are the hot bath to induce perspiration, hot compresses and foot and arm baths to reduce inflammation and pain, and contrasting hot and cold baths to quicken circulation and body reaction. While a *hot* hand bath allays pain and spasm in the hands, a *cold* bath can be used when the body is over-heated, or to control a nose bleed.

Steam

Steam is available by boiling water, using a vaporizer or humidifier, or utilizing either home or professional steamroom, or sauna, installations. Steam increases skin action and creates perspiration, which in turn cleanses the body from within. Steam facials open the pores and keep them clean, and can help prevent skin problems and acne. Hot steam from a vaporizer eases chest congestion. Cool moist air from home humidifiers adds moist air to dry winterized rooms, thus preventing nasal and sinus conditions, and eases a great many airborne allergic problems.

Knowing the correct water treatment, and knowing how to use it, can save you needless pain and expense, and help you to take more active control of your health.

The preceding introduction to the basics of water therapy gives only a glimpse of the vast range of medical uses to which water can be put. In the following chapters we will explore in much greater detail, and with step-by-step, carefully illustrated directions, more than 500 ways that you can use water to improve your health, and to maintain good health for you and your entire family.

(2)

The
Useful
Past

Water therapy is as old as man himself, and it is ironic that such a natural, effective medicine has to be rediscovered in each era. One of the first written mentions of the use of water as medicine involves the temples of the Greek god of medicine, Asclepius. At the temples, bathing and massage were part of the treatment for the sick. Hippocrates, whom we consider the "Father of Medicine," is alleged to be a descendant of the legendary Asclepius. Hippocrates used water as a beverage in reducing fever, and for treating many diseases. He also stressed the value of using various types of baths, each with a different temperature, as a therapeutic tool to combat illness.

Later, the ancient Roman physicians Galen and Celsus also advocated specific baths as an integral part of their remedies. A series of cold baths are known to have cured the Roman Emperor Augustus of a baffling disease that had resisted all other remedies, and thereafter cold baths were much in vogue in Rome.

Almost every warm-climate civilization has at some time used baths for therapeutic reasons as well as for pleasant social interaction. There is an interesting medical footnote on the great Persian physician Rhazes, who was the first to comment on the difference between measles and smallpox. Rhazes wrote on the action of perspiration in forcing the eruptions to quickly emerge. This concept is very important in water therapy, and has been known and used by physicans in India, Turkey, Russia, and Finland, as well as by the medicine men of the American Indians.

Throughout history there are indications that water was used as a remedy in controlling high fevers, but the remedy was so simple that its use waned as other modes of treatment were introduced. It is interesting to note that during the eighteenth century there was a great revival of the use of water as medicine among some Italian, German, and English clergymen, and that the dedicated Scottish physican and surgeon, Dr. James Currier, wrote an important book, *The Effects of Water, Cold and Warm, as a Remedy in Fever and Other Diseases.* Currier detailed his clinical use of cold water drinking and dousing to reduce high fevers, particularly in typhoid and smallpox, and his use of cold water for its internally stimulating and reactive powers.

Currier wrote his first book in 1797. However, it was not until the early nineteenth century that Vincent Preissnitz, a Silesian farmer, laid the foundation of modern water therapy. Vincent was only a teen-ager when he first became interested in water's healing powers. He had mangled his fingers and, as he watched with amazement, a neighbor showed him how to use continuous, wet cold compresses to cure and restore the function of his injured fingers. Shortly after this episode, Vincent was loading hay into a cart on a hill when the horses bolted and the heavy cart rolled over his body. To all appearances Preissnitz was crippled for life —at least that was what the doctor told him. But Preissnitz remembered the lesson of his fingers. He daringly forced his caved-in ribs into a more natural position, and again tried cold compresses to relieve his pain. The combination of rest, copious water drinking, and wet cold wrappings worked beyond his wildest dreams. He fully recovered and water therapy was "invented" once again.

History is studded with such isolated medical successes, but what is really extraordinary is that this teen-age farmer took his own experience with a therapy and developed it into a whole therapeutic system. Preissnitz's cure was so spectacular that he immediately won the respect and interest of his fellow villagers. Because he had so many varied health problems to work with, Preissnitz was able to *experiment* with folk remedies, concepts that strangers brought to him from other lands, and his own variations. And since he was tenacious and analytical, he developed many new techniques for using water: single or double compress packs, dousings, full and partial immersions and, of course, those famous cold "douches"—streams of water which we call showers.

Word soon spread of this extraordinary farmer who could perform miracles with water. Hundreds of sick people came from all parts of the Austro-Hungarian Empire and, under the direction of Preissnitz, each house in the village of Grafenberg was transformed into a miniature spa. Although his system won many followers, it also provoked great controversy among practicing physicians who eventually took Preissnitz to court. He not only won his case, but the leading physician of the Empire, Baron Turkeim, came to observe his methods, and reported to the Emperor that they worked. Thereafter, Preissnitz was under the protection of the Crown, and visitors came to him from every land.

One of these visitors, an English disciple, Dr. Erasmus Wilson, noted that Preissnitz was able to devise these simple, yet intricate techniques *"because his mind wasn't cluttered with the medical impossibilities of such an achievement."*

Preissnitz did not write down his procedures—rather they were written up by literate men or physicians who came to observe his system. He had a startling impact on English, German, and some Scandinavian, as well as American, disciples, but it wasn't until Sebastian Kneipp that water therapy became truly international.

Kneipp was born in 1821, in Bavaria, a few years after Preissnitz. He was a weak and frail youngster who was determined from early childhood on to become a priest. However, repeated illnesses interfered with his studies and activities. During one of his many long convalesences, he chanced to read a pamphlet; we do not know yet whether it was one by a religious colleague, or one about Preissnitz. The pamphlet discussed the use of cold water to strengthen the body and make it disease-resistant. The concept electrified him. Although it was the heart of the Bavarian winter, he went to the river and plunged in. Determined to strengthen himself, he repeated this icy plunge every day, and in a short time he became markedly stronger. He developed extraordinary stamina, vigor, and strength, which he maintained through a long and active life as a priest. Cold water and water therapy made him the renowned Charles Atlas of his day.

Kneipp shortened some of Preissnitz's techniques, and also developed strengthening concepts of walking either in cold water, or on wet grass. We owe the next set of innovative hydrotherapy procedures to his clinical activities.

Kneipp was also a practicing herbalist, and he combined many herbal therapies with the water techniques. Among his most important contributions was the use of such inexpensive herbs as hayflower or oatstraw for detoxification purposes. He experimented with healing procedures for a great many diseases, and was particularly active in helping to heal children. He developed the wet "nightshirt," dipped either in salt water or hayflower water, and this was one of the keystones of his treatment for children's diseases.

After Kneipp, many prominent English, German, and American scientists investigated the therapeutic action of water on the body. I am indebted to these scientists, physicians, and lay persons who continuously observed and noted the clinical action of water on children and adults who recovered from acute or chronic conditions as a result of hydrotherapy.

PART II

Water Ways: Techniques in Using Water for Therapy

The Medical Uses of Water

Water's three forms—liquid, steam, ice—can be used in a wide variety of *temperatures* and, especially in the case of showers or whirlpool, can be used with different *pressure.* Water can be used *internally* by drinking it, or by forcing streams of water into orifices, as in an enema, douche, bidet, or nose or ear bath. And water can be used *externally* in the form of full or partial baths; showers, even on minute spots of the body; single or double compresses, or various body compresses or packs; hot water bottles; frozen ice bandages, or wrapped ice; steam in several different ways; and various simultaneous or alternate combinations.

Because water can be used in so many ways, it has an astonishing variety of health uses. The following are the *general* therapeutic uses of water:

As a Restorative and Tonic

Water not only restores the body's normal circulation and temperature, but intelligent water treatment, especially with cold water, can also act to restore and increase muscle strength, and increase the body's resistance to disease.

Cold water boosts vigor, adds energy and tone, and aids in digestion. *Techniques:* Cold water treading, whirlpool baths, cold sprays, alternate hot and cold contrast showers or compresses, salt rubs, apple cider vinegar baths, salt baths, partial packs.

For Injuries

The application of an ice pack will control the flow of blood and reduce tissue swelling in most injuries.
Techniques: Ice bag, plus compression and elevation.

To Relieve Pain

Even when drugs fail, an application of direct moist heat alleviates nervous irritability and reduces pain. Both hot and cold applications may be used to either reduce inflammation, act as a counterirritant, or divert blood to other areas.

Techniques: Hot and cold compresses, ice bags, warm or hot baths, hot packs, enema, paraffin baths, whirlpool baths, hot and warm or alternate hot and cold showers. *Do not use heat on a fresh injury:* it increases blood flow and inflammation, and therefore tissue swelling.

For Minor Burns

Water, particularly cold and ice water, has been rediscovered as a primary healing agent for minor burns, such as grease, candlewick, and hot glass burns.

Techniques: Ice water immersion or saline water immersion.

To Reduce Fever

Water is nature's best cooling agent. Unlike drugs, which usually only diminish internal heat, water both *lowers* the heat and *removes* it by conduction. In reducing fever, water is far more valuable than any medicine, and it is the treatment of choice for fever, sunstroke, and heatstroke.

The Brand Cold Bath technique, or cold baths, should be reinvestigated as adjunct therapy in typhoid and typhus fever.

Techniques: Short cold baths, prolonged tepid baths, dousings, sponging, cold mitten massage, high enema irrigation, damp sheet packs.

To Induce Perspiration

The skin is the largest organ for elimination, and simple immersion in a long hot bath or a sauna or steamroom visit can stimulate excretion of toxins from the body through the skin. The inducing of perspiration is useful in treating acute diseases and many chronic health problems.

Techniques: Hot baths, epsom salt or common salt baths, hot packs, dry blanket packs, hot herbal drinks.

As a Diuretic

The application of water can effect kidney action to increase urine production as high as 100%, and can also help maintain the normal pH balance of the urine.

Techniques: Ice water for drinking, diuretic herbal teas, hot moist compress applied to lower back, various cold sprays, alternate hot and cold sprays, cold trunk pack, sauna, full and partial blanket pack, and other perspiration inducing therapies.

As an Eliminative

Water is a *perfect* eliminative agent. It can dissolve excrement as well as foreign elements of the blood through irrigations and through induced perspiration through the pores of the skin.

Techniques: Warm water colon irrigation, genital irrigation, drinking water, kidney stimulation applications, vapor, sauna, or hot baths, damp sheet packs, dry blanket packs, hot moist packs.

As an Antiseptic

Boiling water can be used to cleanse food and clothing in viral and bacterial diseases.

Techniques: Immersion in boiled and then cooled water, immersion in chamomile or calendula (pot marigold) steeped tea, cleansing with soap and water.

As a Laxative

Drinking water is generally necessary for proper elimination of waste materials, and can be used for specific laxative and purgative effect to flush material from the bowels.

Techniques: Two glasses of cold water on arising, enema.

As an Emetic

It sometimes is necessary to eject poisons (viral, food, etc.) from the digestive system.

Techniques: Drink copious amounts of warm water, salt water, or mustard water. No other vomiting agent is needed.

To Raise Body Temperature

Hot water transmits heat and warms the body.

Techniques: Hot full baths, hot water bottle, hot foot bath, salt blanket packs, cold friction massage.

As a Stimulant

Water applications can revitalize, awaken, or arouse parts of the entire body.

Techniques: Hot or cold baths, sponging, damp sheet packs, enema or colon irrigation, whirlpool baths, salt rubs, salt baths, hot or cold showers, alternate hot and cold showers.

As an Anesthetic

Water can dull the sense of pain or sensation.

Techniques: Ice to chill the tissues.

As a Sedative

Water is a very efficient, nontoxic *calming* substance. It soothes the body and promotes sleep.

Techniques: Hot and warm baths to quiet and relax the entire body, salt baths, neutral showers to certain areas, damp sheet packs.

As an Antispasmodic

Water effectively reduces cramps, and can help overcome both hysterical and infantile convulsions.

Techniques: Chamomile enema, cold water or hayflower dipped shirt, hot compresses (depending on the problem), herbal teas, abdominal compress.

Water therapy does not replace the need for immediate medical care in the case of convulsions.

To Relieve Thirst

Drinking copious amounts of water assuages the thirst and restores the alkalinity of the blood.

Techniques: Drinking pure (glass bottled) water, distilled water with lemon juice, water plus fruit juice.

For Buoyancy

Bedridden patients will feel better, and avoid bedsores, when the body is buoyed by special "strip" water mattresses. In burn centers, badly burned patients are placed in tubs of sterile water so that nurses can gradually remove the burn scabs. Temporarily disabled or paralyzed accident victims, and those with severe muscular and skeletal problems, always feel better and move better when immersed in a pool of warm water. Often those who cannot walk at all may be able to move freely in water because of the buoyancy.

Techniques: For bedsores: water mattresses, and frequent sponging. For muscular or skeletal rehabilitation: use the physiotherapy facilities in your local hospital, as electric equipment is necessary to deliver the patient on a stretcher into the pool.

For Mechanical Effects

Different pressures of water can exert a powerful mechanical effect on the nerve and blood supply of the skin.

Techniques: Friction rub with sponge or wet mitten, dousing, streams of hot or cold water directed at various parts of the body.

TYPES OF WATER APPLICATION FOR HEALTH PURPOSES

Water can be used in many different ways depending on the health need and condition of the patient, as well as the facilities available for therapy. Among the most effective techniques are direct *localized* applications, water streams, full or partial baths, sponging or other friction techniques, steam for cleansing and detoxifying, neutral washings, wet cloth wrappings, or cloths impregnated with various healing substances. A special water therapy technique devised in the early nineteenth century is a cold compress or pack with a dry outer wrapping which creates internal heat.

Local heat: Apply heat to specific area of the body such as joint, chest, throat, shoulders, spine. Use hot moist compress, hot water bottle.

Local cold: Apply cold to a specific area of the body. Use cold compress, ice bag, ice pack, ice hat, frozen bandage.

Cold compress that heats the body: A cold wet cloth covered with a dry cloth, or a water resistant covering, will create internal heat, and warm up the area from within. This is called the cold double compress. It can be applied to any area of the body, or used as a complete body pack.

Tonic friction: Water sponging, and washing combined with some form of *friction,* from a hand to a rough wash cloth, produces a tonic effect in the body. Use cold mitten massage, cold sponge rub, wet sheet rub.

Sponging: Use alcohol or water or witch hazel applied to a sponge to wash the body.

Baths: The body is immersed in cold, hot, or tepid water. Use foot baths, sit baths, full baths, herb baths, or pharmaceutical baths. Any part of the body may be partially bathed, as in arm bath, eye bath, finger bath.

Pack: A pack is a larger form of the double compress, or may consist of a poultice of clay, flaxseed, or mustard. An example is the hot blanket pack, damp sheet pack, hot leg or hot hip pack, mustard pack, mud pack.

Showers: Several kinds of water streams can be directed against the body. Alternate streams can also be directed against the body, or large quantities of water can be poured from a height. Use dousing, jet, fan, or alternate hot and cold Scots shower.

Shampoo: When soap and water are used together on one or all parts of the body, it creates a shampoo. Use to cleanse hair, or after sauna or steam room.

Steam: A vaporizer can cleanse the upper respiratory system, and a steam room or sauna increases body perspiration and releases many stored toxins. Cold steam, as from a humidifier, moistens dry rooms in winter and is important in preventing colds and sinus headaches.

GENERAL AREAS OF THE BODY

To Help This Area	Use Water Therapy on Skin in This
BRAIN	Face, scalp, hands, back of neck
PHARYNX and LARYNX	Neck
Mucous Membrane of NOSE	Back of neck, hands
LUNGS	Chest—front and sides, across shoulders
HEART	Nerves around the heart
LIVER	Lower right chest
SPLEEN	Lower left chest
KIDNEYS	Lower third of breastbone (sternum), lower dorsal and lumbar spine
STOMACH	Mid-dorsal spine
INTESTINES	Lower dorsal and lumbar spine, abdomen, especially umbilical region
PELVIC ORGANS (ovaries, bladder, rectum)	Lower lumbar and sacral spine, shoulder, lower abdomen, groin, upper inner surfaces of thighs, from navel to breast bone (center)
HANDS	Head (brain), mucous membrane
FEET and LEGS	Brain, lungs, pelvic organs
LOWER ABDOMEN, GROIN, and Upper Inner THIGH	Pelvic organs
UTERUS	Spine of lower back, lower abdomen, inner surface of thighs, breast, feet
BLADDER	Inner surface of thighs, feet, lower abdomen

Drinking Water

Drinking water is such a natural and necessary activity that we tend to forget that it also has many health functions. Whenever you feel sick, it is a good idea to greatly increase the amount of water you are drinking. I know that when I feel sluggish or overtired I tend to crave large quantities of two of my favorite bottled waters: Evian and Mountain Valley Water. Both are pure, taste good, and have excellent mineral ingredients.

Filtering Water

The question of pure water is an urgent one throughout the world. I keep a carbon filter on my kitchen tap, and I feel that it does help to filter out some impurities, especially chlorine. If you intend to use such a filter, remember to *change it* often. Although these filters will take out some gross impurities, they cannot filter out carcinogens, and an alarmingly high percentage of local waters contain toxic and disease-producing chemicals.

Bottled Water

Should you use bottled water? In some states, such as California, a large percentage of people buy their drinking water in the supermarket.

17

But I have discovered that some bottled waters in America are only reconstituted, distilled, or deionized tap water. Also, water is often sold in plastic bottles, which sometimes leech their petrochemical base into the water. This defeats the purpose of buying bottled water. Glass bottles are a safer choice, but be careful choosing what brand of water you buy. Some of my favorites are Mountain Valley Water, Evian, and Perrier. Other good brands are San Pellegrina, Poland Water, Fiuggi.

Allergy to Water

Lately, physicians have noted the fact that many people are increasingly *allergic* to their local water. Most patients never realize that it is the water that is causing their mild bouts of depression, slight or major headaches, diarrhea, or even arthritis. Various allergists report that as many as 50% of their patients are sensitive to local water, and prescribe one of the eighteen or so international and local pure mountain or spring waters.

Because this is such an important problem, I list in the Resource List in the Appendix (page 230) a national distributor for many of the top bottled waters around the world. Perhaps, like Michelangelo, you will discover a bottled water that will help you overcome a specific health problem. In 1559, he drank the Italian water, Fiuggi, and it helped him to overcome a kidney stone problem.

Some naturopaths prescribe demineralized, *distilled water* which can be obtained by the gallon from drugstores. Because of the absence of minerals, such water is said to act as a cleansing magnet by attracting unnecessary minerals in the bloodstream. Distilled water is alleged to be helpful in arthritis as well as some other health problems. *However, the absent minerals must be replaced through food intake or through judiciously selected supplements.*

Drinking Water Therapy

Some of the many health problems that respond favorably to drinking water therapy include: fever, diabetes, rheumatism, arthritis, constipation, common colds, gallstones, edema, smoking, alcohol drinking, drug intake, digestive problems, athletic cramps. See also individual listings of health problems in Part III.

Fever: Drinking 2–3 pints of cold water (about 40°F) can reduce a high fever from one-half to two degrees in ten minutes.

Cold water lowers temperature, absorbs the heat of the fever, and dilutes the blood. It also helps the skin and kidneys to eliminate the very toxins that have caused the fever reaction. It also increases evaporation of fluids and this also reduces the fever.

Fever patients should drink from 6 to 8 quarts a day.

Diabetes: Diabetic patients should drink copious amounts (6 to 8 glasses a day) of pure water and fluids to remove, via the skin and kidneys, all the unoxidized sugar from the body.

Rheumatism-arthritis: It is helpful for rheumatic and arthritic patients to drink large quantities of water in order to dissolve and eliminate uric acid and other waste materials, and to stimulate skin and kidney function.

Constipation: Drink 2 glasses of cold water before breakfast to help overcome constipation.

Common colds: Folk wisdom, as well as orthodox medical practice, advises drinking "lots of fluids" before the onset of a cold, and during such an attack. Drinking pure, room temperature water, and copious amounts of hot herbal teas, will flush the system and help to restore normal functioning.

Gallstones: Drinking 8 to 12 glasses of water a day will greatly dilute the bile secretion, and flush the liver.

Edema: When the tissues of the body—especially in the feet—are swollen, it is necessary to drink several quarts of pure water a day. But it is advisable to drink it only early in the morning and in the evening—*not* in the intervening hours. If additional water is necessary, drink it in ounce quantities only.

Smoking: Heavy smokers should drink copious amounts of water to eliminate the cigarette toxins from the body and to stimulate the liver in its detoxification activities.

Alcohol drinking: Drink copious amounts of water to flush the alcohol from the system and to help the liver eliminate the foreign toxins deposited by the alcohol.

Prescription drugs: It is helpful to drink copious amounts of water while on a regimen of prescription (or hard) drugs. This flushes the drug out of the system after it is "used," and helps the liver detoxify the substances.

Always take yogurt, or acidophilus tablets or liquid, when on a prescription drug. This restores the necessary intestinal flora, helps more normal elimination functioning, and may help to prevent a yeast infection following long-term drug use.

Digestive problems: Drinking cold water acts as a tonic to the digestive system, but it is hot water that aids and relieves chronic gastritis, hyperpepsia, and colic.

Drinking Water, Fluids, and the Athlete

Professional and Olympic athletes know that they must drink water consistently in order to perform well. That is why many athletes travel with cases of their favorite bottled water, or have it sent on ahead to every training camp and game. Muhammad Ali always drinks the French water, Evian, in this way.

Drinking water has an important role in sports. In normal life, we must drink a certain amount of water simply to exist, but this amount must be greatly increased when we engage in sports, especially competitive sports. This is due to the 2–3% body water depletion in such activity, and also because internal water intake affects both *calf cramps* and the *fatigue level* of the body.

Sports physicians note that it takes about ten playing days in hot weather for the body to accommodate its salt conserving capacity and therefore advise athletes to drink large quantities of water before, and during, every playing break. They also advise *adding salt*, either directly to the drinking water in the amount of a one-half teaspoon to a quart, or by swallowing 2–3 salt tablets, and flushing them down with large amounts of neutralizing water. Such salt replenishes the supply excreted through urine or sweat, and greatly *lessens* the possibility of *heat prostration*. A former professional baseball player, amateur boxer, and jujitsu teacher, Dr. Jose Rodriguiz, feels that such salt and water intake also helps in the necessary production of adrenalin and sometimes "acts like magic" in sports.

Dr. Rodriguiz also notes that before-game abdominal jitters are often helped with an increase in the drinking of acid drinks, such as tomato juice. *Avoid* taking *antacids* for such spasms, he urges, since such substances contribute to the perpetuation of the cramps.

In addition to salt-laced water, or high potassium drinks, such as organic vegetable soups, etc., *herb drinks* are useful. *Chamomile* tea will also reduce stomach spasms and quiet the body, *linden* tea will quiet the nerves and help ensure restful sleep the night before a game, and *peppermint* tea is delicious, refreshing, and stimulating, and is easily prepared in large quantities and served cold before, during, and after games.

Cayenne pepper, in very tiny doses, will also help to settle digestive rumblings, and provide a small boost in energy. For digestive disturbances, add a few *grains* of the powdered cayenne pepper to a hot herbal tea: chamomile, peppermint, or linden are excellent. For energy, add a tiny pinch or several grains per glass, or about ¼ teaspoon to a quart of pure *grape* juice, and sip as needed.

Drinking Water for Newborns

I have often been asked if newborn infants should be given purer water than the adults. The answer is definitely yes. The newborn child is susceptible to dehydration, and needs water that is almost mineral and sulphate free. Because infants are susceptible to gastrointestinal upsets, it is also very important to have a water source that has a low bacteria count, and no toxic deposits. Certainly, in the first weeks, the infant needs help in getting the kidneys to function normally, and fresh, pure water is essential in activating kidneys, causing perspiration, and maintaining internal heat balance.

If you live in an area with a poor water supply, or high mineral and high sulphate content, you should definitely use one of the better bottled waters. Evian bottled water, highly regarded by French mothers and their physicians, is available throughout the United States.

As the baby grows, it should drink the same water that you drink, except in exceptional circumstances of illness or severe diarrhea (see page 138.) In these cases, use bottled water again.

Ice

Ice has a numbing effect, and therefore immediately reduces the discomfort of strains, sprains, contusions, hematomas, and even fractures. The cold also acts to control any internal hemorrhage by reducing the fluid build-up in the body tissues.

Ice also has a *secondary* use in later *rehabilitation* of injury, and for chronic spastic conditions. Ice helps to increase the range of motion, stimulates the muscles, and decreases spasticity and pain. Ice massage or ice bath or indirect applications are used in such rehabilitation by physiotherapists. This speeds the early return of the patient to normal or athletic activity.

Acute Injury

There is uniform agreement that *heat must never be applied to any acute injury.* Heat has the opposite effect of cold. It increases blood flow, and the metabolic rate, and thus increases the inflammatory response and production of tissue fluid. These are negative responses in acute trauma.

Ice, on the other hand, decreases the amount of pressure in the capillary vessels and lowers the extent of the bleeding into the tissue spaces. Cold decreases the body temperature of a particular area. This slows the total metabolic process within the cells of that area, and consequently lessens the cells' need for oxygen and nutrients. This reduction in metabolism results in a reduction of the swelling.

Another important benefit of the periodic application of ice is the prevention of hematoma—a tumor or swelling which contains blood. This is often the result of severe body impact such as occurs in sports or in accidents. When ice is applied immediately following injury, and continued as described (see the alphabetical list of health problems in Part III), the probability of pain and edema—the retention of fluids in tissues —is also diminished.

Wrapped Ice Bags

A wrapped ice bag is the most effective *initial* therapy for most injuries, especially sports injuries. An ice bag is a waterproof rubber container. It comes in different sizes and for different parts of the body, and is available at most drugstores. If you cannot obtain an ice bag, you can achieve somewhat the same effect by wrapping ice in a towel.

Most specialists prefer to use ice in an ice bag which is in turn lightly wrapped in a dry cloth, and attached to the injury site with an elastic bandage to keep it slightly squeezed. This *compression* reinforces the physiological action of the cold application.

In order to avoid frostbite or freezing, place a layer of fabric between the skin and the ice bag (the wrapping on the ice bag will do). The injured part is then immobilized by bed rest or elevation. The three related injury procedures are easily recalled with the acronym I-C-E which represents the words *I*ce, *C*ompression, *E*levation.

The total length of time for ice therapy varies by injury and severity, and possibility of recurrent hemorrhage. Most professionals use ice bags plus compression in *20–30 minute sessions, usually two times a day.* (In my experience cold is most effective in 20 minute segments.) But sometimes

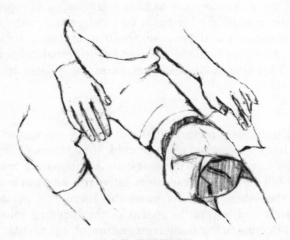

I.C.E. THERAPY

Fig. 1.   I.C.E. stands for Ice, Compression, and Elevation. Ice therapy controls bleeding, lessens pain, and reduces swelling. It is useful in athletic as well as other injuries. For knee or other injuries, first protect the skin with an intervening fabric, and apply ice in an ice bag or in a towel. Attach the ice with an elastic bandage to create a slight compression. Elevate the area.

shorter applications are desired, up to four times a day. Most injuries respond within the 24–48 hour span, while some require up to 72 hours of periodic ice attention. Specific details as described by some noted team physicians, coaches, and trainers are given in Part III.

Frozen Bandage

I use these homemade frozen bandages for minor sprains, minor first aid, and the release of such spasms as do not respond to moist heat. See pages 24–25 for the method of making such a bandage.

ICE BAG
(soft waterproof rubber container holding ice)

THERAPEUTIC USES

Stop bleeding	Relieve joint pain
Relieve pain after injury	Reduce head congestion
Numb an area	(apply to head)
Check congestion	Protect heart during heat
Prevent swelling in sprain or	application on other parts
contusion	of the body
Check inflammation	or for heart problems

An ice bag in a leakproof rubber container is one of the most useful and versatile of water therapies. It is also one of the several possible cold applications to the head—the others being ice turbans and "hats," ice packs, cold compresses, and sponging with ice water. Always start these applications with tepid water. (See further details for cold applications to head on page 24.)

To fill an ice bag, first get rid of the sharp edges of the ice, or somewhat crush the ice. For a head or chest application, fill the bag half full. If the back of the neck or the head is to *rest on* the bag, fill the bag completely. In either case, expel the air before screwing the lid. Make sure to fasten the lid very tight. First, dry the bag (a wet bag can freeze the skin) and cover it with a thin kitchen or hand towel. The covering is important as it makes the initial reaction less intense, and also prevents the body from heating up the bag (the reverse of what you want to accomplish). For this reason, it is important to replace the ice as soon as it melts because it then changes into a warm compress.

Do not apply cold continuously, but rather periodically. Also, rub the part of the body briskly with the hand between applications of ice.

ICE PACK
(ice in a towel)

THERAPEUTIC USES

When ice bag is not available
When ice application is needed for large body area
As a cold application around the entire neck
As a turban for the top of the head

When packing a joint to reduce pain, or avoid swelling in
   injury

Empty about 3 freezer trays, crush the ice, and place in the center
of a large, folded bath towel. This can be applied as an ice collar around
the neck, or around a joint, or as a large ice application to other parts of
the body. Use an intervening layer of fabric to protect the skin. Massage
the skin frequently to reinstate reactive powers and prevent freezing of
the tissues.

ICE TURBAN

Ice turbans are made by soaking a large, light towel in ice water and
winding it around the head. Place crushed ice in another small, porous
towel, and apply over turban to the top of the head. Ice packs have the
same action as an ice bag where the ice is enclosed in a rubber container.

COLD APPLICATION TO HEAD
(bag, towel, cold cloth)

THERAPEUTIC USES

Eliminate fatigue of the body or mind
Prevent or control headaches
Control faintness
With other applications for a loss of memory, worry,
   depression
As cold compress during hot foot bath, or any hot moist heat
   application to the rest of the body
During attempts to induce perspiration

There are various kinds of cold head applications including ice
"hats," ice packs, ice bags, and cold compresses. Short applications are
very tonic, and excite mental activity, as well as helping to decongest the
head. Long applications of cold to the head will lower the temperature
of the brain, and lessen internal vital activity as well as production of heat.

When cold compresses, packs, or turbans are used during perspira-
tion-producing therapy, renew the compresses every few minutes, otherwise they become warm compresses. Also stabilize the procedure by
increasing the intake of drinking water. This replaces the fluid lost with
excretion of toxins.

FROZEN BANDAGE

THERAPEUTIC USES

Minor sprains   Spasms that don't react well to heat
Minor athletic injuries   Some sciatic tension

I always keep several of these handy ice aids in my freezer, as sometimes the body takes more kindly to these bandages than ice. They are
invaluable when you need to marshal internal heat within the body.

Unlike ice bags, which stay continuously cold, frozen bandages gradually become warmer and warmer. Children love being treated with these special bandages.

Method

Plunge a dish towel in ice cold water. Wring out the water. Fold towel lengthwise, and in half. Insert into a plastic bag. Place the bag, or bags, in the freezer on a piece of cardboard so that the cloth will freeze flat.

To use, pull off the plastic, and apply to the body. As internal heat rushes to the cold area it will soften the stiff bandage. Soon the bandage will conform to the body area. For a sciatica attack that doesn't respond to moist heat, place an intervening cloth and lie down on the frozen bandage. Often two consecutive bandages will eliminate the spasm.

Compresses

Cold water, hot water, or liquified medications and herbs can be applied to any area of the body by means of folded cloths called compresses. These are created with either cotton, linen, flannel, or gauze, and are usually in 3–4 inch folds. However, the thicker the folding, the longer lasting the compress. Because it is lightweight and easily available, a linen or cotton dish towel is usually my favorite choice for an instant compress, but sometimes larger cloths are needed.

Three Kinds of Compresses

There are three kinds of compress applications.

Hot: Single or *double.* Sometimes called a *fomentation* (a relaxant).

Cold: Single (inhibits circulation, flow, bleeding).

Double (stimulates circulation). This compress consists of one wet cloth completely covered by a dry cloth.

Alternate hot and cold: Sedates and then stimulates.

Area Compresses

Compresses are frequently named for the *area* they are to be applied to—for example, head, throat, joint, chest, trunk, foot, genital, or hemorrhoidal. Since many of these area compresses consist of *large* cloth wrappings, they can also be called *packs.* Most packs are actually double compresses.

Health Problem Determines Choice

The health problem that needs to be solved determines the compress temperature, duration, and whether or not herbs should be added to the water.

COLD DOUBLE THROAT COMPRESS
(a heating compress)

Fig. 2.   A double compress consists of a *cold wet* cloth covered with a larger *dry cloth.* This is one of the unique and remarkable techniques in water therapy, the paradox being that a cold application will heat up and relax the area. This is achieved by the outer, airtight covering which actually traps the heat delivered from within the body.

The cold double compress may be used in various shapes and sizes on any part of the body. The large body compress is based on this concept. The triangular compress (Fig. 5) and the chin-ear compress (Fig. 4) are also cold double throat compresses.

Apple cider vinegar water may be used instead of plain cold water.

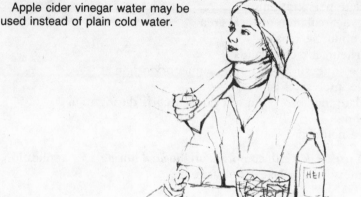

Adding to Compress Water

Apple cider vinegar can be added to either hot or cold compresses —*except those applied near the eyes or genitals.* When adding vinegar, use a tablespoon to half a cup in the compress water. For hot compresses, add the vinegar to the water being heated. Vinegar detoxifies and reduces inflammation. Witch hazel also reduces inflammation.

Other detoxifying substances that can be added to compresses are hayflower, oatstraw, and such healing substances as fenugreek, cooked carrot, oatmeal, raw or cooked onions, baked potatoes (all of which can be used as direct poultices on the area to be healed). In the case of hayflower, oatstraw, and fenugreek, they can be used as *teas* into which the compress cloths are dipped.

A combination of mustard powder and flour plus water can be called a mustard compress, but it is most often called a mustard plaster (or pack). Mustard brings blood to the surface of the skin, and is useful in overcongested areas, as the chest in bronchitis; but it can reduce internal congestion elsewhere as well.

A few drops of a tincture of arnica (arnica being an outstanding pain reliever for unbroken skin) can be added to the compress water while the cloth is being prepared, to assuage pain of *strains* or *sprains.* Use only on *unbroken skin* areas. Sometimes stimulating ointments may be added directly to the skin (again where there are no open cuts or wounds), and the compress is then placed *over the ointment.* Arnica ointment, oil of eucalyptus ointment, wintergreen ointment, or the commercial Olbas ointment are useful for pain. Calendula (pot marigold) ointment can be applied directly to the skin under a compress in the case of sores, cuts, or prior bleeding.

HOT MOIST COMPRESS

THERAPEUTIC USES
   Relieve pain
   Stimulate perspiration
   Improve circulation of local area
   Relieve muscle spasms
   Help rheumatic complaints
   Reduce congestions of noninflammatory origin
   Relieve intercostal pain
   Stimulate the absorption of cellular debris during injury
      healing
   Relieve neuralgia

Always use a *cold* cloth compress on the *head* during a *hot* application. Hot, moist heat relaxes contractions.

Time Used

Long applications of 30 minutes to a maximum 2 hours are *sedative.* They are thus useful for spine and sleep problems.
   Short applications of 3–5 minutes are *stimulating.*
   The effect of consecutive applications of hot moist cloths is similar to a vapor bath, paraffin bath (antipain), or an old-fashioned mud pack at a spa. As the hot moist cloths are replaced, that area of the body is alternately heated and cooled. This relieves the muscle spasm.

Sciatica, Internal Spasm, Colic

My father always said there was no better treatment for sciatica than a series of long hot-compress applications, each followed by a *short* cold shower. Actually, all rheumatic problems, muscular pain, lumbago, and pain under and around the breast are helped by hot moist compresses. These applications can be repeated every evening until the problem disappears. In the case of gallstone colic or intestinal colic, or for relief of spasms or painful period, apply a trunk compress every half hour.

Polio Breakthrough

Sister Kenny discovered the value of hot moist compresses during a 1920s polio epidemic in Australia. Desperate to relieve the pain of her patients, she remembered the water therapy her family had used when she was a child. She kept renewing the packs which were left on for 12 hour periods. Most of her patients recovered the use of their limbs be-

HOT MOIST COMPRESS
(fomentation)

Fig. 3.   Hot moist heat lessens pain, muscle spasm, and neuralgia and also helps rheumatic complaints. Use old wool or soft cotton. Fold the cloth in three parts and refold into a narrow strip. Dip the center of the cloth into boiling water. Twist and wring out ends. Carry in cloth carrier in order to retain heat. Renew fomentation as soon as it loses heat.

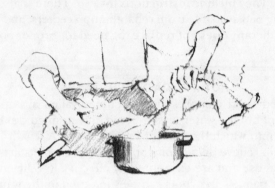

cause she stretched and reeducated the muscles every hour after the heat application. These hot compresses prevented the muscles from shortening.

Method

In advance boil water, and have several cloths ready for immersion before each treatment. Use an electric hot tray to keep the water boiling, or else keep the previously prepared hot cloths *covered* in a blanket. You can carry several of them in a pail covered with either a hot water bottle, a blanket, or newspapers.

Old wool is not irritating to the skin and provides the very best material for long-lasting hot moist compresses. However, large cloths of soft cotton or linen can be used.

Fold each cloth into three, and then refold into a narrow strip. Fold this strip in half so that you can hold the edges in one hand while you dip the center into boiling water. Twist tightly by the dry ends. Next, pull the ends apart. This helps to squeeze out the water. It is important *not* to use a dripping wet cloth! As soon as the cloth is squeezed out, place in the dry cloth "carrier" and carry to patient. Several such cloths are needed.

If the skin is sensitive, stroke oil on it, and stroke the area. Apply the hot cloth in a rocking manner, holding up one end and lowering the other. If it is still too hot, put your palm under the cloth and stroke the skin again. This relieves the heat impressions and partly cools the area at the same time. Do not lift the cloth up as this may chill the patient.

Cover the hot wet cloth with a dry towel.

Have the next hot moist compress ready before removing the first.

In *very* acute attacks of pain, as in muscle spasms, renew the hot compresses every few minutes. In most acute attacks they can be renewed at 15 minute intervals, or as soon as needed, but on the whole, hot compresses can be left on from 30 minutes to 2 hours.

When there is a need for frequent hot moist application to relieve pain or muscle spasm, purchase silica gel hydrocollator applications from the drugstore. They include instructions for use. There is also a wet-heat electric heating pad available from rehabilitation centers, and some drugstores. Water therapy does not replace the need for proper polio vaccination.

HOT MEDICATED COMPRESS

A hot medicated compress is sometimes called a stupe. An herb dissolved in hot boiling water or simmered and strained can be added to the hot water into which the cloth is being heated. A few drops of *arnica tincture* will help relieve pain. Homeopathic arnica tablets are also available for internal use and are exceptionally effective in relieving muscular and rheumatic pain. *Ginger* roots can be simmered in the water and then brought to a quick boil before the cloth is immersed, or ginger powder can be dissolved into the boiling water for pain relief.

Many of the most famous spas in America such as the Golden Door envelop their guests in herb-dipped body wraps, actually the equivalent of large body compresses. These wraps, which usually include a small amount of wintergreen and eucalyptus and other herbs, can help to reduce pain and bring blood to the surface of the skin.

Another method of applying medication with moist heat is to apply pain relieving *ointments* such as arnica, Olbas (a commercial product), wintergreen, or eucalyptus *directly* on the unbroken skin, and then cover the anointed area with a larger hot moist compress.

When it is desirable to bring blood to the surface, use a thin paste of mustard powder, flour, and water. (See Mustard Pack, page 93.)

Apple cider vinegar may be added to either hot or cold compress water.

COLD SINGLE COMPRESS

THERAPEUTIC USES

Prevent headaches (use on head or neck)

Help prevent congestion of heart area (use on heart area)

Anti-inflammatory

Reduce temperature of body, or part of body

Reduce blood flow to local area

Relieve pain

Prevent swelling in injury

Relax during crying jag

A cold compress acts in an *inhibitory* fashion. The thicker the fabric, the longer the cold will last. The initial effect of the cold is contraction; then, as the internal reaction warms the area and the cloth, the flow of blood helps to break up deeper seated or nearby congestion, as in an injury or inflammation.

If there is a possibility of a neuralgic effect, apply a light cloth between the skin and compress.

Method

To make a single cold compress, fold a cloth (the size depends upon the need for which it is being used) in half or thirds. Dip it into either cold tap water or ice water. Wring it out thoroughly and apply. Renew cold compresses every few minutes to keep the cold constant.

To reduce even further the possibility of swelling, and to reduce pain of a sprain or strain, you may add a tablespoon to a half cup of either *witch hazel* or *apple cider vinegar* (*no vinegar near the eyes, of course*) to the compress water. Apple cider vinegar is also detoxifying. *Hayflower* water made with prepared extract, or from a handful of the flowers steeped in a quart of boiling water and strained, may be added to any compress to increase the detoxifying action and reduce swelling. Such hayflower compresses wrapped around the feet and legs will reduce swelling of feet.

All three of these herbal substances act in an extraordinary fashion. Keep each on hand to experiment with. Witch hazel is sold in drugstores, apple cider vinegar is on the grocery shelves, hayflower bath extract is noted in the Resource List.

Weleda sells Luvos Earth #2 for compresses, and the Three Sheaves Company sells French green clay for compresses. These are used cold or hot in a cloth or applied directly on the skin. See Resource List.

In cases where constant cold is needed for longer periods—as in sports injuries, abrasions, contusions, hematoma, sprains, strains, initial fracture (until professional help arrives)—use an ice bag, or crushed ice in a plastic bag. Keep a towel between the skin and ice, attach with elastic bandage to provide needed compression, and elevate the injury as described under each problem in Part III.

Temperature of Compress

Temperature: 42°F–60°F is considered very cold.

Higher compress temperatures needed for weak or frail patients: 70°F–85°F.

Compresses to heart area: About 60°F.

Usually, the colder the application, the briefer the application should be. See specific health listings in Part III for details.

Duration of Compress

Time: 10–60 minutes. Renew every few minutes. Massage the skin under the compress every 15 minutes to help the body to react properly to the cold.

Use up to two times a day, or more often when specified.

COLD DOUBLE COMPRESS
(wet cloth, covered by dry cloth of flannel or wool)

THERAPEUTIC USES

Acute joint inflammations	Hemorrhoids
Chronic arthritis	Gastrointestinal problems
Pneumonia	Sore throat
Insomnia	

Congestive headache } Renew every few minutes.
Hayfever

Tonsilitis }
Ear infections
Acute laryngitis }
Diphtheria
Croup
Measles }

1. In early stage renew every 2 minutes to inhibit inflammation (single compress).

2. Follow by double (wet plus dry) stimulating compress to bring blood to area. Renew every 30 minutes, or when dry.

Note: This compress has a general *heating* effect, as do all cold double compresses (abdominal, genital, throat, etc.).

The cold wet compress, covered with a piece of dry flannel or wool, is the invention of Preissnitz, and is an extremely effective self-care tool. The double throat compress, the one you will probably use most often, is especially helpful in upper respiratory infections. Since these compresses are applied to one local area at a time, they improve the circulation in that area, increase elimination from that area, improve local nerve function, assist in the discharge of internal catarrh, and also work on the reflexes to the central nervous system of the part of the body to which they are applied.

COLD DOUBLE THROAT AND EAR COMPRESS

THERAPEUTIC USES

Sore throat (neck compress)
Earache (neck and ear compress)
Tonsilitis (neck compress, neck and ear compress, or triangular compress)
Mumps or swollen glands (neck compress or neck and ear compress)
Bronchitis (triangular compress)
Pneumonia (triangular compress)
Influenza (triangular compress)
Asthma (triangular compress)

Note: This compress has a general *heating* effect.

There are three different double compresses for the throat, neck, and ear region. Each is made in the same way, but is wound around the neck in a different direction.

Neck Only

This compress is used mainly for sore throats, and may be combined with either the ear or triangular compress. This compress can also be used for tonsilitis, swollen glands, or mumps.

Method

Fold a cotton dish cloth or piece of a sheet in thirds. Dip it in cold water, or diluted or full strength apple cider vinegar. Wring out. Wind *once* around the neck and fasten with a safety pin. (Optional: Wind a plastic bag over the wet cloth.) Over the wet cloth, or cloth and plastic, now wind a large *wool* sock or wear a wool dicky. Make sure no air intrudes.

This is one of the most effective and important water therapies. It works as follows: The cold compress is "trapped" by the larger, warmer one, and the throat and neck are warmed internally. This provides warmth and increased circulation which work together to help conquer the sore throat. It also works well on laryngitis.

Neck and Ears

This compress was invented by the renowned hydrotherapist Dr. Simon Baruch. It is excellent for mumps, swollen glands, and earaches.

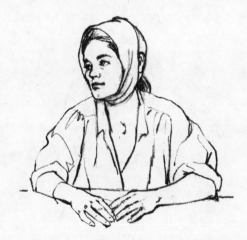

COLD DOUBLE THROAT AND EAR COMPRESS

Fig. 4. This ear winding was created by Dr. Simon Baruch, an advocate of scientific hydrotherapy and an early exponent of the holistic approach to health. The compress is effective for ear problems, swollen glands, and sore throat.

Fold a narrow cotton cloth in half or thirds. Dip in cold water or apple cider vinegar water. Wring out. Pin around the neck. Repeat the process with a slightly wider cloth, and wind around the chin to the top of the head. Pin. Make a slit for the ears. Cover the neck with a piece of plastic or brown paper and pin an old wool sock over it so it is airtight. Cover the chin to head with another piece of old wool or nonporous cotton.

Method

Follow the same procedure as for the neck compress. Wind the compress as above, but then wind *again* from the chin past the ears to the top of the head. Make a slit in this second compress for the ears. Tie or pin on top of the head.

Triangular (for neck and chest)

This is a neck compress plus a partial chest compress. It is useful in helping combat tonsilitis, bronchitis, pneumonia, influenza, and asthma.

Method

Apply the neck and partial chest compress as below. Then, in addition, cover the wet compress with a larger dry kerchief or a wool dicky so that this second compress extends over the chest.

To sum up: These above compresses may be used somewhat interchangeably, depending on the area that needs warming up. The important thing is that the first compress (winding) must be cold and wet. It may also be dipped in any of the herbal preparations mentioned for detoxification, especially apple cider vinegar. The outer cover must be

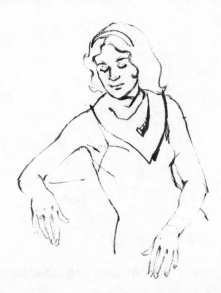

COLD DOUBLE TRIANGULAR THROAT COMPRESS

Fig. 5.   A kerchief-style compress covers the entire throat as well as part of the chest, and is useful in throat and chest complaints. It consists of two cloths. Dip the first cotton triangle in cold water or apple cider vinegar water. Wring out. Apply around the neck. Cover the area with a larger, nonabsorbent dry cloth. It is sometimes helpful to protect the wet layer with a piece of plastic or brown paper. This helps to trap the heat emanating from the body in reaction to the initial cold application. All cold *double* compresses produce heat.

wool to keep out the air. In an emergency, a second layer of brown paper (from a brown paper bag) or a large strip of plastic can be used underneath or instead of the wool outer layer.

A cold double throat compress will not only overcome laryngitis, but will help cure most sore throats. This technique is also effective in relieving earaches. I was traveling in England and Scotland recently, and not unexpectedly the weather was extremely rainy and chilly. I suddenly developed a slight earache which, to my later regret, I ignored. That night, however, the pain awakened me from a sound sleep.

Since I was traveling and didn't have compress materials, I was initially at a loss. Should I tear up a towel or a pillow case, I wondered? I finally settled on tearing up my husband's white cotton undershirt. After wetting the strips with cold water—they proved to be limp but serviceable —I carefully wound them first around my neck, and then from the chin to the top of the head. I used a turtle neck sweater for a throat cover, and wound a wool sock over both ears, and a scarf over the sock to insure airtight fit. I looked like a Martian with mumps, but no matter, I slept soundly and awakened completely free of the earache. Despite continued inclement weather, that was the last of that ache.

COLD DOUBLE CHEST COMPRESS

THERAPEUTIC USES

Bronchitis	Influenza	Pleurisy
Asthma	Pneumonia	Emphysema

Note: This compress has a general *heating* effect.

A double, stimulating compress applied to the chest area, or wound over the front and back, is a most useful aid in overcoming breathing problems. This compress can ease a deep-seated cough, and generally improves the circulation of the chest area.

Method

First method of application: Dip a flat cloth or medium-size bath towel into cold water. Wring out so that it is slightly dripping. Apply to chest. Cover with a larger dry towel. This loose arrangement gives immediate access to the chest, and the wet cloth can be replaced by another cold one every few minutes, or cold water can be gently sprinkled onto the bottom towel. This quick replacement is necessary in very acute upper respiratory attacks.

Second method of application: Apply a wet cold compress in the form of a criss-cross bandage over the chest and back. Cover the wet bandage with a large, form-fitting wool sweater. Lift off the sweater and sponge the wet bandage with cold water every 30 minutes. Alternate another dry sweater as a cover. When doing this, the patient must lift his or her hands, and change position and sitting arrangements. This contributes to the healing process. *Make sure that the patient does not become chilled.*

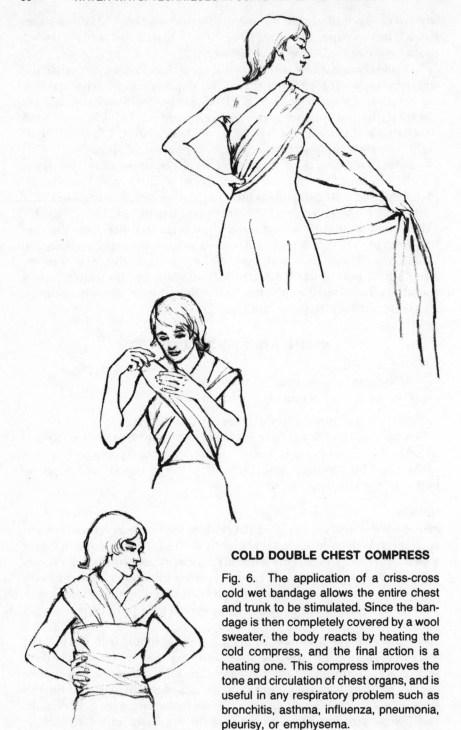

COLD DOUBLE CHEST COMPRESS

Fig. 6. The application of a criss-cross cold wet bandage allows the entire chest and trunk to be stimulated. Since the bandage is then completely covered by a wool sweater, the body reacts by heating the cold compress, and the final action is a heating one. This compress improves the tone and circulation of chest organs, and is useful in any respiratory problem such as bronchitis, asthma, influenza, pneumonia, pleurisy, or emphysema.

Third method of application: Use two large towels. Dip each in cold water. Wring out. Place protective material on bed. Apply half of one towel to back, half of other towel to back. Fold each over the chest area. Cover with large dry towels.

COLD SINGLE TRUNK COMPRESS

THERAPEUTIC USES

High fever
Hemorrhages: liver, pancreas, spleen, stomach, intestines
Preliminary treatment to other treatments

It is sometimes urgent to inhibit certain actions within the body, such as a high fever or internal bleeding. A cold single trunk compress can be used in these cases.

Water therapy does not replace the need for immediate medical care in the case of internal bleeding.

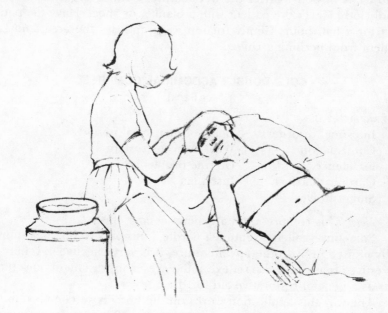

COLD SINGLE TRUNK COMPRESS

Fig. 7.   A cold water application to the trunk of the body will help reduce fever or internal bleeding. Double or triple fold a terry towel or large cotton cloth, dip into cold water or apple cider vinegar water, and wring out slightly, but apply rather wet. To prevent chilling, cover with a light cotton blanket, and make sure the room is warm and draft-free. Renew the compress every half hour or when the cloth is dry or warm. Also see Abdominal Compress and Chest Compress, and reflex points for this area of the body.

Method

A cold single compress can be made from a large double or triple-folded towel, or from a folded cotton sheet. Dip the towel or sheet in cold water, wring it out, and apply it to the area between the shoulders and the navel. Cover the patient with a light blanket or large dry sheet. Renew every half hour.

See also the water therapy techniques for treating fever and hemorrhages in Part III.

COLD DOUBLE TRUNK COMPRESS

THERAPEUTIC USES

Chronic pelvic problems   Nervous irritability
Chronic abdominal problems   Insomnia

Method

Fold a large towel in half, dip it in cold water, wring it out, and apply it to trunk of body. Cover the wet compress with a larger dry towel or wool cloth. Cover the patient with a blanket or sheet. Have the patient rest for a half hour. Gently friction wash and dry the area, and keep patient from becoming chilled.

COLD DOUBLE ABDOMINAL COMPRESS
(or Pack)

THERAPEUTIC USES

Intestinal disorders   Delay of menstrual period
Constipation   Weak nervous system
Flatulence   Uterine problems
Chronic diarrhea   Insomnia
Sluggish liver

Note: This compress has a general *heating* effect.

Sometimes called "Neptune's Girdle," this pack technique is universally praised in hydrotherapy literature. It is very effective in toning the digestive organs, and also reflexly influences many distant organs. It thus acts as a general restorative aid for the body.

The way this application works on the body is so complex and interesting that it deserves special explanation. The combined wet and overlapping dry compress diverts a large amount of the blood to the skin of the trunk and the portal circulation section of the body. The portal system is capable of holding most of the blood of the body. When the blood is diverted, it causes a contraction of the cerebral blood vessels, and creates a tendency to sleep. This hypnotic effect takes place almost at once—unless a chill sets in, in which case it doesn't work at all.

Method

Use about 3 yards of light, coarse toweling. Wet half of the toweling with tepid water, wring it out until it stops dripping, and apply to abdomen, placing one end at the side, and bringing the rest across the front of the body so that two thicknesses of wet towel cover the abdomen. Wind the rest snugly around the body, and fasten. *For feeble patients, wet only that portion that touches the abdomen.*

Cover the entire wet portion with a flannel cloth and fasten. Change the wet bandages every 30 minutes. Between applications, wash the abdomen with cool water, and lightly friction dry the area.

In acute cases, where a high fever is present, change the wet bandages every 30 minutes. Remove the compress when dry. Friction sponge the abdomen, and dry with light friction strokes.

In treating chronic digestive problems, the compress may be left on the entire night, and removed the next morning. Cleanse the abdomen with cold water, and friction dry. This compress is also helpful in overcoming chronic *insomnia* cases.

In the past century, before the introduction of antibiotics, this water therapy was highly praised by physicians for its ability to help cure appendicitis, and particularly typhoid fever.

Since certain preferred antibiotics no longer respond to the typhoid bacillus, this technique may be of great importance once again. It can also be used as a prophylactic measure to tone the body during typhoid epidemics.

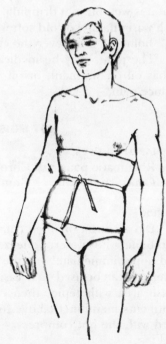

COLD DOUBLE ABDOMINAL COMPRESS
(or Abdominal Pack)

Fig. 8. "Neptune's Girdle" has been used for over 130 years to restore body tone in the abdominal area. This cold wet abdominal compress is attached over the stomach area and covered with a larger airtight cloth. It can be effective in digestive disturbances, insomnia, uterine problems, nervous system problems, and with delayed menstruation.

COLD SINGLE JOINT COMPRESS

THERAPEUTIC USES
Acute joint inflammation   Ulceration   Scalding

Method

Fold a cloth about the size of a dish towel several times. Dip it into cold water. Wring out the cloth so that it is wet, but not dripping, and lightly fasten around the inflamed joint. Since the pain may be intense, do not disturb the compress, but lightly sprinkle cold water on the area every 15 minutes in order to keep the compress continuously cold. To treat burns or ulcerations, add vitamin E oil or ointment of the juice of the aloes plant after the acute attack is over, and apply the following cold double joint compress as secondary therapy.

COLD DOUBLE JOINT COMPRESS

THERAPEUTIC USES
Chronic arthritis, or nonacute attacks (wrist, hand, knee, ankle, foot)

Note: This compress has a general *heating* effect.

Method

Dip a long, narrow compress cloth into cold water, wring it out so that it is wet, but not dripping, and bind spirally around the joint. Cover with warm flannel or old soft wool, and fasten. Change every 30 minutes to 2 hours, or whenever the compress warms up and dries.

The joints may be medicated first with arnica lotion or ointment, Olbas oil or ointment, or oil of wintergreen to increase circulation or reduce pain.

HOT MOIST JOINT COMPRESS

THERAPEUTIC USES
Rheumatic pains   Chronic joint problems
Contracting skin   Gout

Method

Dip a cotton or linen compress that has been folded several times into boiling hot water. Squeeze out the water until there is no dripping, and apply immediately to the area of joint pain. To relieve pain, this compress can be used on occasion, or several times a day, six hours apart. Wash area with tepid, then cool water, and friction dry. The herbal ointments mentioned above for the cold double compress may also be used with the hot compress.

GENITAL OR HEMORRHOIDAL COMPRESS

Method

Use either *hot* or *cold* compresses. To overcome pain and *sedate* the area, use *warm* or *hot* moist applications. To reduce *inflammation* and tissue disruption, use *cold* applications. Both kinds of compresses work by acting on the local group of nerves feeding the sympathetic system of the area.

COLD DOUBLE GENITAL COMPRESS

THERAPEUTIC USES

Rectal inflammations	Inflammation of the
Inflammation of the anus	scrotum or testes
Prolapse of the rectum	Inflammation of the prostate
	Inflammatory hemorrhoids

Note: This compress has a general *heating* effect.

Method

Attach a cold compress with a T-shaped bandage, or sanitary pad belt, and cover the wet compress with a dry flannel cloth. In acute attacks, change every 15 minutes until relief occurs.

For chronic rectal or genital lesions, renew the cold compress every hour, or when warm and dry. It may be left overnight.

HOT MOIST RECTAL OR HEMORRHOIDAL COMPRESS

THERAPEUTIC USES

Rectal straining during evacuation
Spasms in certain hemorrhoidal conditions
Straining of the bladder during urination
Painful spasm of the vagina.

Method

Fold a linen cloth the size of a dish towel into thirds. Dip it into hot water. Wring it out, and attach it, using the same method as with the cold double compress. Renew every half hour until spasms stop, or area is sedated.

COLD SINGLE FOOT COMPRESS

THERAPEUTIC USES
Pain relief

Method

Fold a large towel into thirds. Dip it into cold water and wring it out. Apply to area of pain, either folded on top or wound around the foot. Replace cloth often so that the area is constantly wet and cold.

GENITAL OR HEMORRHOIDAL
COMPRESS
(hot or cold)

Fig. 9. For inflammatory genital or hemorrhoidal problems, use a *double cold*
compress. (Apply a cold compress and
cover it with a dry cloth.)

For rectal, vaginal, or bladder pain or
spasm use a *hot* compress and renew
every half hour.

Both the hot and the cold compress affect the local nerves feeding into this area.

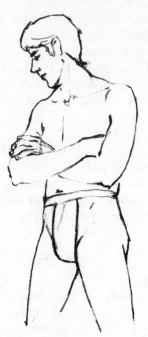

COLD DOUBLE FOOT (WET SOCK) COMPRESS

THERAPEUTIC USES

Overcome and draw heat from another part of body

Overcome exhaustion

Decongest head passages during bad cold

Relax entire body

Decongest lungs, chest, and bowels

Note: This compress has a general *heating* effect.

Foot compresses are a very effective old country remedy. They were
my grandmother's favorite way of overcoming the discomfort of a bad
cold. The compress takes only an hour or two to be effective, but it can
be left on all night. As it unclogs the closed nasal passages, the patient
relaxes into a quiet sleep.

Method

Dip long strips of cloth into either cold water or water diluted with
up to 50% apple cider vinegar. Wring out the cloths so they are wet, but
not dripping, and wrap them in spiral fashion on the feet and legs. Wrap
dry bandages *over* the wet compress.

An easier method is to dip long cotton *knee socks* in cold water or
vinegar-water, wring them out, and pull up over each leg up to the knee.
Pull long dry wool socks over the wet ones. Cover the feet with an
additional blanket. After the initial chill, the area will warm as the blood
congesting other areas (i.e., head, chest, abdomen) rushes to the cold
expanse at the lower part of the body.

COLD DOUBLE FOOT COMPRESS
(or Wet Sock Compress)

Fig. 10.   This is old country magic for overcoming the annoying effects of head congestion or a cold. This technique also helps to overcome body exhaustion and produces a night of serene sleep.

Dip a knee-high cotton sock into cold water or apple cider vinegar water. Wring out. Apply immediately to each foot. Pull on a long wool sock and *completely cover the wet area.*

If no long socks are available, use strips of cotton, cover with plastic or brown paper, and tie on an airtight, nonporous cotton or wool cloth.

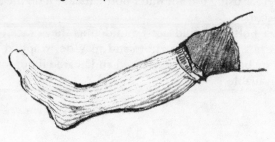

HOT SINGLE FOOT WET SOCK COMPRESS

THERAPEUTIC USES

    Spasms of the foot   Excessive callus   Neuralgia

Method

    Pat the feet with light cream or vaseline. Dip long cotton knee socks into very hot water. Wear rubber gloves to wring out socks, and immediately apply to each foot. Change every 2–3 hours.

HOT WATER BOTTLE

THERAPEUTIC USES

    Create instant warmth and comfort   Sedate and relax an
    Intensify any other heat   area
      application   Increase perspiration
    Relieve menstrual cramps   Relieve sinus attacks
    Alleviate pain

    In the old days, people used hot bricks and copper warming pans to transfer heat to the body. Nowadays we have flat, portable, and inexpensive rubber containers. Hot water applications must sometimes be dry, yet have the penetrating quality of moist heat, and the hot water bottle meets this need. A hot water bottle will relax the body, reduce spasms and pain, and hasten the healing process by absorbing cellular debris. It is a versatile health tool that should be in every home.

    A friend who is a writer tells me that he uses a hot water bottle over the forehead, and over the bridge of his nose to relieve the pain of a severe sinus attack. A hot water bottle can be wrapped in a towel and applied near the abdomen of a colicky child. Or it can be used along with loud ticking clocks to relax puppies who are away from their mother for the first time. Hot water bottles can also be used to warm cold feet and to relieve severe menstrual cramps. Several hot water bottles can be used together to stimulate a sluggish heat reaction in a feeble, exhausted, or comatose patient.

Fill the rubber bottle three quarters full with hot—never boiling—water, and wrap it in a towel before applying to any area of the body. If you have sensitive skin, apply either a vegetable oil or easily absorbed cold cream before using the hot water bottle. Leave it on the affected area until relief occurs.

Hot water bottles should not be folded as they crack.

Hot salt, hot cornmeal, or hot sand may be wrapped in a double pillow case, or a bread may be decrusted and heated if hot water containers are not available.

(7)

Baths

I am addicted to baths. I like them cold, hot, and neutral. Baths are pleasure rituals, as well as for health and cleanliness. In addition, the right bath, and there are many to choose from, is effective, inexpensive medicine.

Many ancient cultures used baths for ritual and health. The actual custom of bath chambers may have been created by the Egyptians, and then improved upon and developed by other cultures living on or around the Aegean Sea. Bathing was also an integral ritual in Jewish tribal life. Even in the Dark Ages, when the Church frowned on bathing, the Jews maintained public bath houses. This may be one reason this small group survived the decimation of the bubonic and other plagues.

The ancient Minoans left the remnants of bathing apartments in the palaces of Cnossus and Tiryns, as did the very ancient Greeks who created luxurious bathing areas complete with heated water, cold showers, and plunging pools. We know from the fragments of medical history passed on by word, and in writing, that the eminent Greek physician Hippocrates advocated the use of baths as medicine. As one of the early and great clinical observers he noted a direct correlation between the use of partial and full baths, and healing in many diseases. Hippocrates was one of the first physicians to state that nature should be used to heal the body; he realized that the body's capacity for self-healing was so strong that nature needs only a boost to start the healing process.

My own favorite baths vary with mood and according to need. I like hot water baths to relax and soothe the body, and to overcome aches and pains. However, long hot baths deplete the energy and tone within the body. Cold water, on the other hand, restores body tone. In the case of pain, or when you want to relax before sleep, or if you wish to produce perspiration to eliminate toxins, bacteria, or disease from the body, warm or hot baths are effective. Otherwise, use either neutral, cool, or cold water baths. For tonic effects there is *nothing* better than cold water. No matter what your own bathing preference is, remember to end each bath and shower session with *cool or cold water.*

To improve your energy level, vitality, and disease resistance, use the cold treading bath, or a version of that cold bath, every day.

FULL COLD BATH

THERAPEUTIC USES

Stimulates the body	Lowers extreme fever
Acts as a tonic	from disease or
Promotes resistance to disease	heat attack

Short Full Cold Bath: For *healthy* persons

A cold plunge into very cold water is an exhilarating experience. I had my first experience with the use of the cold plunge after a sauna in Stockholm. The first effect was a slight shock to the body, then *complete pleasure.*

Method

To duplicate the famous Swedish cold bath at home, first warm your body up with hot drinks (herbal teas are excellent), a hot steamy bath, or hot steamy shower, and then immerse your body in a *full tub of cold water* from the tap. The first effect is chill, followed by comfort. A second chill will follow, however, so leave the bath very soon after you feel the comfort set in. Always end this bath with a vigorous towel rub.

Remain in the bath for 30 seconds to 2–3 minutes, depending on your tolerance. Many people who use this bath develop such a tolerance that they can remain several minutes longer.

This bath produces a sense of deepened vitality. All the famous American and European spas encourage clients to take this plunge after steam and/or sauna sessions since the cold plunge completely revitalizes the body.

Do not use this bath if you have organic diseases, high blood pressure, nervous temperament, or if you are weak, very old, or very young, or have heart weakness, colitis, or hardening of the arteries, as in these cases the body's reaction is usually negative.

The bath temperature should be below 65°F (18.3°C).

Prolonged Cold Full Bath: For *ill* persons

THERAPEUTIC USES

High fever	Typhoid
Heat prostration	Typhus

"Cold bathing is a power for good, before which all other measures must stand aside," said Dr. H. A. Hare of this antifever treatment, sometimes called the *"Brand Bath."*

Method

First warm the patient with either a hot drink, hot shower, hot moist compresses, hot water bottle, or other warming method. Then gently splash the patient's face with cold water.

Carefully lower the patient into *cool* water, 65°F–75°F (18.3°C–23.9°C). With the hand, *constantly massage the patient to keep the blood on the skin.* Or massage can be accomplished by wrapping a damp cold sheet around the patient before he or she steps into the bath. The *sheet* is then slapped and rubbed constantly to create additional friction. The patient should remain in the bath only a few seconds. This is also called a *wet sheet* bath.

Dr. Brand's cold immersion bath was developed in 1861 during a typhus epidemic. Since then, the bath, combined with *constant massage,* has saved the lives of many typhus and typhoid victims.

This bath should only be used in dire emergencies, as it is a great shock to the body.

FULL HOT BATH

THERAPEUTIC USES

Alleviate pain

Reduce muscle spasms

Relieve internal congestion

Induce perspiration

Eliminate fatigue after exercise (short)

Relax and calm the body

Hot baths are useful to sedate and relax the body, to relieve pain, and to eliminate toxins from the body through the skin. They can also be used to warm the body for other cold water therapies. I use hot baths (sometimes with herbs and medicinal substances added) after exercises or to help abort a cold. However, hot baths deplete energy. Make sure to apply a cold compress on the forehead to offset the rush of blood from the head (depletion).

Method

Fill the tub completely. Start running the bath water at body temperature, or slightly higher, and gradually increase the water temperature until it is as hot as the body can tolerate comfortably.

Position the body so that the head is resting comfortably against a small rubber pillow or rolled towel, and all parts of the body are completely submerged. Apply a cold compress to the head and keep it there for the duration of the bath. Remain in the bath for 2–20 minutes, depending on comfort and need. As the bath water begins to cool, let a little out and replace it with hot water from the faucet. Do this as often as necessary to maintain the desired temperature.

If the bath is to induce perspiration, do not add cool water, but get out of the tub, wrap body completely in towels to avoid being chilled, and immediately get into bed under blankets (or follow with technique for "damp sheet compress," or hot blanket pack).

If the bath is *not* for the purpose of detoxification or inducing perspiration, end the bath by gradually letting out all the hot water and replacing it with cool water. As a final step, splash cold water all over the body. Get out of the bath and dry the body by rubbing it vigorously with a heavy towel.

Short Full Hot Bath

A two minute hot bath is similar to cold application and helps when recovering from exhaustion after exercise. A short hot bath eliminates metabolic fatigue, and stimulates nerve centers.

Prolonged Full Hot Bath

A longer hot bath, from 20–60 minutes in duration, is the water therapy for arthritis, gout, gall bladder, neuralgia, bronchitis, and the relief of muscular fatigue.

It is never to be used by very old, very young, weak, or anemic persons, or those with severe organic diseases or a tendency to hemorrhage.

TONIC FRICTION BATHS

The action of a cold water *massage* with hands or *friction* materials such as sponges, hand mittens, or loofah has a profound *tonic* effect on the body. Cold bathing plus friction stimulates and creates a circulatory and heat response within the body. All tonic friction techniques are invaluable for bedridden or weak patients.

There are four tonic friction baths: sponge bath, cold mitten massage bath, brush bath, and salt massage bath.

SPONGE BATH

THERAPEUTIC USES

For weak patients	For insomnia
When body is overheated	Whenever water is needed for
To reduce fever	medicine

This is the simplest of the friction baths, as it generally requires only several quarts of water. (In emergencies, as little as one pint of water can suffice.) Remember that a *warm* sponge bath sedates; a *cold* sponge bath stimulates.

Method

Splash the face with lukewarm water. Dip the sponge in water (or water to which a small amount of apple cider vinegar has been added), and sponge the body in sections, keeping each part of the body warm or covered. Salt or sodium bicarbonate can also be added to the water.

Rub the skin vigorously with the sponge until the skin is fairly red, moving from the upper part of the body to the lower. Be sure to rerub the upper part at intervals to prevent chilliness (especially when reducing a fever).

As soon as the sponging is finished, wind a clean sheet or large towel around the body, and rub dry. Freshen the bed clothes, place a light blanket on the body and take a restful nap.

COLD MITTEN MASSAGE BATH

THERAPEUTIC USES

As a general tonic
To rebuild body stamina
For bedridden patients
For patients too weak to bathe

For people who get colds
  too often
For low blood pressure
To stimulate inactive
  circulation

This is a wonderful bath for bedridden or weak patients as the use of a coarse friction material plus cold water acts as a general tonic on the

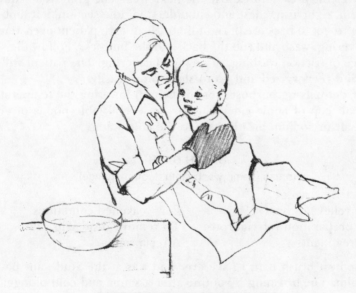

COLD MITTEN MASSAGE BATH

Fig. 11. This sectional friction restores body tone and increases circulation in young, very old, or feeble patients, especially those too ill to bathe themselves. This massage reduces fever and is an effective self-help aid for people who are susceptible to colds.

The body is covered except for the area to be washed. Rub the uncovered area with a rough mitten or rough wash cloth dipped into cold water or apple cider vinegar water. Wipe vigorously to create additional friction. Cover the area and repeat massage on another part of the body until the whole body is washed and massaged.

This friction massage can be used by well persons to achieve a feeling of well-being. (For another effective tonic friction, read section on salt massage.)

body. The consistent use of this simple "sectional" bath, with only one part of the body available for friction or air at a time, improves the blood's circulation. This, in turn, promotes the process of internal self-healing.

Method

Cover the body completely, and only *expose one small area at a time.* Start the process by gently splashing the face with cold water. For exceptionally old or weak, or heart patients, it is also beneficial to apply a cold compress to the head, and an ice bag on the heart area. This allows the circulation to remain within the other parts of the body.

You will need a pan of cold water, several towels, and two towel mittens, towel holders, or hemp wash cloths. Put on the mittens, or hold a pot holder in each hand, as the two *simultaneous* friction movements increase the tonic reaction. Dip each of the mittens in the pan of cold water, and start by stroking the right arm, rubbing and washing at the same time. As soon as you are finished rubbing, vigorously rub the area dry. Cover the area, and expose the next area. The preferred sequence is left arm, right arm, chest and shoulders, middle section, left limb (lift each leg to get to back area), right limb. Next, turn patient over, remove back covering, wash and rub the back and the buttocks. Follow the same sequence of friction washing, drying, and covering. The patient will feel rested and reenergized and go to sleep more easily.

For detoxifying purposes, or for help in lowering the temperature, add a half cup of apple cider vinegar or several tablespoons of either coarse salt or sodium bicarbonate to the cold water.

BRUSH BATH
(brush, hemp wash cloth, loofah sponge)

THERAPEUTIC USES

To relieve asthma	For weakened conditions
As preparation for vigorous treatments	To remove dead skin cells
	After a sauna

The best brush bath I have ever had was at the Studevant Bath in Stockholm. The brushing is routine after a sauna and cold plunge, and acts like a combination massage, deep pore body cleanser, and body tonic.

This bath may be used for invalids, or used by healthy people to remove dead skin cells.

Method

Soap the entire body with a nonabrasive, emollient soap or avocado oil. Dip a large non-nylon brush, hemp wash cloth, or loofah into hot water, and scrub the skin for 2–5 minutes in circular motions until the skin is red and the body feels invigorated. End the bath with a warm shower, gradually reducing the water temperature until it becomes cool.

SHALLOW BATH
(Sit or Sitz Bath, or Hip or Half Bath)

THERAPEUTIC USES

Note specific therapeutic uses under *each* temperature and
bath duration

A *shallow, sit* (sitz is the German word often used to describe this
technique) bath is a bath of 6–8 inches of water, up to the buttocks. A
hip or *half* bath extends to the hips and partially up to the lower abdomen.
These baths have a profound physiological effect on the body because the
hot, cold, or tepid water acts only on a localized section of the body. A
sitting or kneeling cold bath, used daily, will help build resistance and
vigor as will several of the cold foot baths.

Method

Immerse only the buttocks, upper thighs, and lower abdomen in the
water. This is achieved by using either a hospital Sitz Bath or a bidet
attachment (see Resource List), or by sitting in an ordinary bathtub in 6–8
inches of water with legs either elevated on a rubber pillow or elevated
and *wrapped in hot towels,* or covered with a blanket. Sometimes the feet
are immersed simultaneously in a hot foot bath. This speeds the body's
response to the shallow bath.

During a shallow bath, keep the legs and the rest of the body warmed
by *massage.* Prevent chill to the upper torso by either wearing a shirt or
wrapping the shoulders and upper part of the body in large towels.

Use a cold compress on the head in all *hot* shallow baths.

COLD SHALLOW BATH

Before using any cold shallow bath, first splash face, neck, and hands
with cold water.

Short Cold Shallow Bath

THERAPEUTIC USES

Weakness	Delayed period
Inflammation	Impotence
Constipation	Poor circulation in abdominal
Vaginal discharges	organs

A short cold shallow bath has a remarkable tonic effect on the body.
This bath, and the *cool* shallow bath, may be used every day by normally
healthy persons to increase abdominal tone. Because the bath promotes
internal intestinal movement, it helps to overcome constipation.

For additional abdominal stimulation, rub the abdomen with an inverted U movement in clockwise fashion.

Bath temperature: 50°F–70°F.

Duration: 2 seconds to 2 minutes.

Short Cool Shallow Bath

THERAPEUTIC USES

Constipation	Chronic prostate congestion
Bedwetting	Liver, spleen congestion
Weakness of bladder	Hemorrhoids
Chronic uterine infection	

Add ascorbic acid to this bath to help overcome genital or bladder infection, and promote hemorrhoid healing. Use 1 cup to 5 quarts of cool water and up to one cup of ascorbic acid (vitamin C) crystals.

Bath temperature: 70°F–80°F.

Duration: 5 minutes

Prolonged Cold Shallow Bath

THERAPEUTIC USES

Sedate	Chronic diarrhea	Inflamed
Severe hemorrhoids	Dysentery	prostate

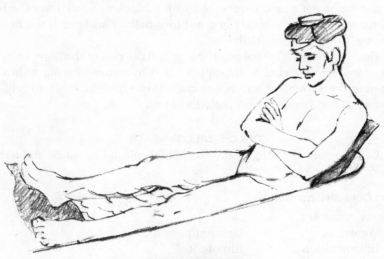

SHALLOW BATH
(or Sit or Hip Bath)

Fig. 12.   One of the miracles of water therapy is its profound effect when directed to only one part of the body (see Hand Bath and Foot Bath). A shallow bath that covers only the lower extremities, in either very cold, very hot, or moderate temperature water, will alleviate a wide variety of symptoms.

Use a cold head compress for any hot application—this is necessary throughout the water therapy system. When possible, elevate the feet by placing them on a rubber pillow. When directed, or if desired, this shallow bath may be taken *simultaneously* with a hot foot bath, or hot foot (or leg) wrappings.

A *cold* shallow bath of a few seconds will help to overcome fatigue, and will invigorate the entire body.

Unlike the short cold shallow bath (tonic) which promotes peristalsis and therefore helps to overcome constipation, a prolonged cold shallow bath (sedative) slows or inhibits peristalis, and will help to overcome severe diarrhea.

Bath temperature: 70°F.
Duration: 10 minutes.

TEPID SHALLOW BATH

Short Tepid Shallow Bath

THERAPEUTIC USES

Quickly lower fever

Bath temperature: 85°F–90°F.
Duration: 15 minutes

Prolonged Tepid Shallow Bath

THERAPEUTIC USES

Sedate
Overcome severe colic

Overcome uterine
spasms

Apply cold compress to the forehead. Start with a water temperature of about 85°F and gradually *increase* the temperature until it is as hot as you can comfortably tolerate.

HOT SHALLOW BATH

Prolonged Hot Shallow Bath

THERAPEUTIC USES

Relieve painful periods
Overcome delayed periods
  (from chill)
Relieve hemorrhoid pain
Relax vaginal spasms
Overcome spastic constipation
Alleviate cystitis (severe)

Alleviate severe sciatica
(half bath, up to
waistline, may also be
used)
Promote perspiration
(half bath may
also be used)

A prolonged hot shallow bath acts quickly to alleviate pelvic area and acute abdominal pain.

During this hot bath, apply a cold compress to forehead, and drink liquids freely. Begin this series of baths with water at body temperature or slightly higher (92°F–98°F+) and gradually over the course of days and weeks develop a tolerance to 120°F. Prevent chilling, keep upper torso completely covered, and conclude the bath with a warm water sponging or shower in which the water used becomes cooler and cooler.

Water temperature in the bath can be increased gradually 1°F by removing one cupful of water and replacing it every 2 minutes with extremely hot water. Each replacement will increase the temperature 1°F.

ALTERNATE HOT AND COLD SHALLOW BATH

THERAPEUTIC USES

Abdominal congestion	Prostate inflammation
Hemorrhoids	Sexual weakness

The alternate hot and cold water produces alternate sedative and reenergizing responses in the body. The general effect is tonic.

Method

Use two separate containers, one with *very* hot water, the other with cold water. First sit in the hot container for 3 minutes, then in the cold container for 1 minute. If it is impossible to use two containers use the same sequence and splash water on the lower extremities. Alternate the hot and cold half a dozen times. Always end with cold water.

For hemorrhoid healing, add several tablespoons of ascorbic acid crystals to each container of water.

WHIRLPOOL

THERAPEUTIC USES

Relieve pain	Remove embedded dirt
Relax spasms	and dead skin cells
Soften scar tissue	Reduce inflammation
Relieve pain after injury	Reduce tissue swelling (edema)
Soften adhesions	Relieve arthritis pain
Increase circulation	Relieve tennis elbow
of the limbs	Relieve knee joint problems
Increase circulation	Alleviate Raynaud's syndrome
within the body	Help parapalegic and polio
	victims

Over the centuries, various cultures have discovered that there seems to be an extra healing force in natural swirling waters. Now, with the miracle of electrical technology we can purchase effective and safe portable whirlpool machines for the bath. We can also duplicate the technique of world-famous spas just by adding minerals or herbs or salts to the water.

There are several whirlpools available commercially, but the most effective and reliable whirlpools are manufactured by Jacuzzi.

One of the outstanding therapeutic uses of the whirlpool is to relieve muscle soreness and fatigue. This is the reason many athletes and dancers purchase portable whirlpools for their bath, or go swimming in a pool with such whirlpool action.

Partial whirlpool therapy is often used by athletic trainers and sports physicians when an athlete incurs a soft tissue injury. First, ice packs are applied to reduce tissue swelling and loss of blood into the tissues and to reduce the flow of blood. The whirlpool is secondary therapy. When possible, the area is isolated so that the whirlpool is directed to the area that needs attention. This usually speeds tissue healing.

Bruce Jenner, the American Olympic Decathalon gold medalist, uses water therapy in this way:

As soon as possible after an injury I put *ice* on it, and continue [this therapy] off and on for 48 hours.
At this point I start whirlpool treatments twice a day; the temperature of the water being 109°F.
In some cases when an injury does not respond I try 5 minutes in the [hot] whirlpool, and use 5 minutes of ice. This [contrast] brings a tremendous amount of blood to the area.

The moving water produced by a whirlpool can relax and at the same time energize the body. Also, because the temperature of the rotating water can be either lukewarm or raised to a very high temperature, whirlpool baths are helpful in antipain therapy. Start the whirlpool bath at a neutral temperature, and raise to the tolerance of the patient. A whirlpool bath can vary from 15 to 45 minutes in duration, depending on the purpose for which it is being used. If you are following the whirlpool with a massage, wrap the entire body so that it stays completely warm.

Whirlpool therapy can help with circulation problems and it is a well-known aid in relieving chronic pain and the phantom pain that occurs after amputations. Whirlpool therapy will help to relieve muscle soreness and body fatigue, especially after vigorous athletic activity. It will also help to heal skin sores and infected wounds, reduce the swelling of chronic edema (tissue swelling), help reduce the pain of minor frostbite, ease scar tissue from burns, and help with weak and painful feet. Many physiotherapists prepare their patients for therapy-massage by first giving them a stimulating and relaxing whirlpool bath.

You can also use whirlpool therapy for Raynaud's syndrome, tennis elbow, knee joint problems, for swollen joints of arthritis, and to improve the circulation of paraplegic and polio victims.

Do *not* use the whirlpool if you are sensitive to very hot water. This includes all persons with diabetes, varicose veins, advanced arteriosclerosis, or any advanced vascular limb problem.

EYE BATH

THERAPEUTIC USES

Reduce inflammation
Relieve sties
Reduce pain on or around eye

Strengthen the eye
Remove foreign objects
  from eye

The eye is very responsive to water therapy. This is partially because the eye is so sensitive, but also because the nerve endings and muscles of the eye can be stimulated directly by water.

Method

Use a sterile whiskey shot glass, or professional eye cup (available at drug stores). Fill with *tepid* water. Apply directly to the open eye and rinse thoroughly.

To strengthen and tone the eye, splash *cold* water on either the open or closed eye first thing in the morning and the last thing at night.

Cold, hot, and medicated compresses will relieve eye inflammation, sties, and pain that generates from the eye area. See the alphabetic listings in Part III for specific instructions.

EAR BATH

THERAPEUTIC USES

Remove hardened ear wax
Remove foreign objects and insects

Reduce inflammation
and abscess

Carefully wash the ear out with a children's syringe. Use tepid to warm water.

HEAD BATH

THERAPEUTIC USES

Sunstroke   Head congestion
Hysteria   Some cases of epilepsy

There are two kinds of head baths:

On Stomach

Place a tub or wide pot on the floor beside a bed. Lie on the bed with the face down and the head extended over the tub. Have tepid water poured on the back of the head from as great a height as possible. Continue until relief occurs.

On Back

Lie on your back with the back of the head resting in a shallow basin of cool water. Have a helper bathe the forehead, face, and temples. Continue this gentle application until the excessive heat is removed or lowered in the body. You may also apply a large folded cold compress to the head and apply the cold water to the compress. This will both intensify the action and keep the area colder.

NOSE BATH

THERAPEUTIC USES

Acute or chronic catarrh

Although nose irrigation doesn't seem natural or easy, it is practiced with great success by those who wish to keep their noses free of pollutants and natural discharges.

Method

Add a pinch of salt to ½ cup of tepid water. Put the water in the palm of your hand, and sniff it up each nostril. This is an effective antiseptic action.

There is a more professional nose irrigation spray that attaches to a Water Pik and may now be obtained for home use. See Resource List, and also "Nose" in Part III.

DROP OF WATER BATH

THERAPEUTIC USES

Inflammation   Wounds   Sprains   Bruises

The capillary action of cotton yarn dipped into water is well known in slow watering of plants. This same ingenious arrangement can be used to cool a wound, bruise, sprain, or inflammation, where the cooling effect is needed for a long time, particularly in the cases where one cannot use ice.

Method

Place a pot with cold water on a bureau or shelf several feet above you. Situate it so that the injured part is directly below the pot. Put one end of a skein of cotton yarn in the pot, and allow the other end to fall over the edge and hang below it. The water will be drawn up into the yarn by capillary action, and drop off at the lower end drop by drop.

PARAFFIN BATH

THERAPEUTIC USES

Arthritis	Local swelling	Strains
Gout	Painful feet	Bruises (unbroken skin)
Sciatica	Bursitis	Tennis elbow
Old sprains	Stiff joints	

A paraffin "glove" is an effective method of delivering high consistent heat to a painful limb or joint. In this process the hand or foot or joint is immersed in, or layered with, a combination of paraffin wax and mineral oil as if creating a thickened series of onion skin. The wax coating raises the internal temperature and relieves the intense pain while creating a long-lasting sensation of pleasant heat. This type of bath was invented in France in the early part of the century, and is used in hospitals by physiotherapists and in many European spas that specialize in the treatment of arthritis. The bath can be created at home in either a double boiler, or with special equipment available from rehabilitation mail order firms. See Resource List.

The instructions for the ratio of paraffin and mineral oil are available from each manufacturer, but usually it takes an hour or more to melt the 2–4 pounds of paraffin wax and 4 tablespoons of mineral oil that are used.

Method

Melt the wax in a double boiler until there is a thin film on the top. Add the mineral oil. Meanwhile, carefully wash the area to be applied. Dip the area quickly into the wax. (If you are treating your hands, keep your fingers separate.) Remove the part until the wax solidifies. Repeat the process until a thick wax glove is formed.

Wrap the affected part in plastic or in a towel. Leave the wax on for 15–40 minutes, and then peel it off. The paraffin can be stored and used again. After a paraffin bath the skin is extremely smooth, soft, moist, and supple, and it is much easier to massage.

In Maine Chance, a noted American spa, women are given *total* body paraffin treatments prior to certain massage therapy in order to completely relax the body.

If using a thermometer, the temperature varies between 126°F–130°F. Do not use a paraffin bath with skin infections, peripheral vascular disease, and any condition of disturbed internal heat or intolerance to heat. Occasionally some persons react to this treatment with a temporary dermatitis.

THE RUBBER HAND AND FOOT BATH

THERAPEUTIC USES

Relieve pain of the hands or feet
Overcome exceptional stiffness of the hands or feet

Anoint the hand or foot with a pain-relieving ointment such as arnica, Olbas, methyl salicylate, or menthol, and place it in a large rubber or surgical glove, or a waterproof bag. Close or tape the glove or bag and plunge the hand or foot into extremely hot water (as hot as you can tolerate). The air layer and the rubber protection allow the limb to obtain a much hotter treatment than could normally be achieved and this prepares stiff or painful parts for massage therapy. (See also "Paraffin Bath.")

This bath may be given every day if needed. The temperature may be as high as 120°F. The bath time varies between 10 and 30 minutes.

Steam

Gaseous state of water is produced by heating water to a high temperature. The wet or dry (sauna) steam is invaluable in stimulating the skin and the resultant perspiration helps to evacuate stored toxins. However, since the water must be hot before it turns to steam it must be handled very cautiously. Test and check each step in any of these suggested procedures to ensure personal safety.

VAPORIZER BATH
(steam from boiling kettle, or electric home vaporizer
or *cold* steam humidifier)

THERAPEUTIC USES

Open pores	Relieve sinus attack
Open clogged nostrils	Relieve head cold
Help breathing problems	Restore voice, overcome
Relieve bronchitis	hoarseness and laryngitis

An 8-hour electric steam vaporizer is a useful home item as it brings moist air into dry, overheated, winterized rooms, and facilitates breathing for all chest and sinus conditions, as well as colds where the nostrils are clogged. It is a big help in a house with children.

Method
Add a few drops of compound or simple tincture of benzoin to the vaporizer lid. The tincture is made from a resin, so it will leave a gummy film, but it is very helpful in chest complaints, and has the added advantage of being a cosmetic aid. It is also a remarkable aid in restoring the voice.

In the event there is no electric vaporizer available, boil water in a kettle, and keep it going by means of an electric tray, or some other safe arrangement. Create an improvised tent over your body and direct the steam so that you don't get too wet or perspired. A large umbrella can be used. Occasionally sponge, or use a cold mitten massage on your body, as this will aid circulation and give a feeling of well-being.

Facials

To duplicate a professional facial, bring to a vigorous boil in a Pyrex pot 2 quarts of water to which 2 tablespoons of chamomile tea have been added. Remove the pot from the heat, place a newspaper on a table, and place the hot pot on the paper. Sit with your face above the pot (but not close enough to get burned). Improvise a tent by surrounding your head and the pot with a towel so that no steam escapes. Sit under the tent with eyes closed for 5 to 10 minutes, breathing with your mouth open. The pores of the face will open and perspiration will pour out. Afterward, gently push out the blackheads with a cotton swab. This procedure is most useful for those with excessively oily skin. Do this in a nondrafty area to avoid chilling. Close the pores with a splash of cool water and sweep face with a cotton pad moistened with an herbal astringent, such as witch hazel.

HOME STEAM BATH

THERAPEUTIC USES

Arthritis	Fractures
Gout	Sprains
Sciatica	Chronic low back pains
Preliminary to tonic cold therapy to eliminate stored toxins	To create perspiration

A free flow of perspiration will often relieve the extreme pain in arthritis, gout, sciatica, and ease other pain. Steam baths are often available in local gyms, and are now available in steamroom or prebuilt sauna units for home use.

A home steam "bath" is relatively simple to construct and basically requires only these extra items: a prebuilt false floor for the bathtub, a long hose from the sink or a short hose attachment in the bathtub, a stool, and a large plastic sheet to create a "tent."

The false bottom should be made of a sturdy, nonsplintering material, and should have sections or perforations for the steam to seep through. It should be elevated 4 inches. Place the false bottom on the tub. Place a stool over the new bottom. Attach a hose to the tub outlet or to a nearby sink. Create a plastic tent over the sides of the tub and your body. Only the head should be out. Open the hot water faucet. The steam will emerge through the bottom sections or perforations. Place a cold compress on your forehead, and use a towel to close any gaps in the tent. Once the routine is established, it may be repeated several times a week provided that you don't get dizzy. The steam may be prepared somewhat in advance. *Be careful not to burn yourself.*

SAUNA

THERAPEUTIC USES

Relieve fatigue	Relieve arthritis
Recover after exercise	Relieve rheumatism
Relieve skin problems	Increase circulation
(chronic eczema, psoriasis)	Eliminate internal waste
Help with menstrual disorders	Increase perspiration
Relieve joint pain	

Many accident victims or arthritis patients find that the dry heat of the Finnish sauna helps them to function in a more normal manner. There is an intense but tolerable heat in the sauna room, and this causes profuse perspiration within a few minutes. The ideal way is to perspire, then take a tepid or a cool shower, and then plunge (if the sauna is at a gym) into a cold pool of water. The total effect of these three water activities creates a feeling of great cleanliness and exhilaration.

The body soon develops a capacity to repeat this process frequently.

Control the tendency for headache or dizziness by applying a cold compress to the forehead.

Portable home saunas are commercially available.

Foot Baths

Ten percent of the total body surface is comprised by the feet. Partial immersion of the feet up to the ankles or calves, in either hot, cold, or tepid water causes reflex contraction in many other parts of the body including the liver, head, and pelvic organs. The body reaction to a cold foot bath is longer lasting than to a hot foot bath.

THERAPEUTIC USES
 For reflex action on other organs
 To cause contractions in other organs
 To divert blood congestion from head, chest, or lower
  organs
 As preliminary to other treatments
 As adjunct to other treatments

 See special details under each type of foot bath.
Types of foot baths: Cold, warm, hot, alternate hot and cold, hayflower, oatstraw, mustard. See also mustard pack (page 93) or Herb and Medicated Baths."

COLD WATER TREADING
(short)

THERAPEUTIC USES

Weakness	Varicose veins	Chilblains
Insomnia	Aching feet	Habitual cold feet
Poor circulation	Nervousness	Catarrhal condition of
Exhaustion	Weak ankles	nose, throat,
		bronchial tubes

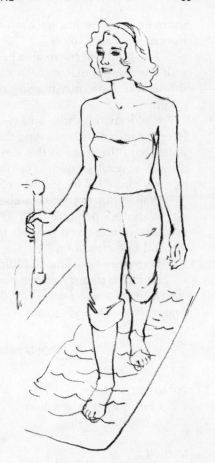

COLD WATER TREADING

Fig. 13. Use this simple water action every morning and evening, every day of your life. It is stimulating and energizing, increases body tone, increases circulation, and helps you develop resistance to infectious diseases. It is an excellent and important procedure for young and old alike.

Immerse feet in cold water up to the ankles, or up to the calves, and move your feet in the water.

I love cold water treading because it produces a feeling of euphoria and good health. Cold water treading, or a cold water whirlpool foot bath, reduces the feeling of heat in the summer and helps to reenergize the body. It is the most important of the *preventive* water treatments because it builds up resistance to disease, and slowly develops a physical vigor within the body. It is no substitute for exercise, of course, but it should be a key part of body care.

Such foot baths help to overcome postexercise leg aches. My jogging friends now take a full warm-hot bath to relieve their muscles, and add a nightly, before-bedtime walk-in-cold-water. They report they no longer have any of the leg cramps that plague many runners.

Method

Fill the bathtub with cold water up to the ankles, or, for a deeper effect, with enough water to cover the calves. Enter the tub, and hold on to a stationary wall grip. March in place for 5 seconds to 5 minutes. In warm or hot weather, walk around barefoot afterward, or wipe the feet vigorously with a towel.

The same effect can also be achieved by sitting on the edge of a tub with a whirlpool motor making a swirling movement in the water, or by sitting and constantly moving the feet and rubbing the soles against a rough surface.

Children, invalids, and postoperative patients can duplicate this effect by sitting and splashing their feet in a large dishpan filled with cold water. Rub the soles of the feet along the bottom of the container. Do this for several seconds. Do not allow weakened or feeble persons to become chilled. The amount of time can be increased week by week.

Walking in wet grass is also strengthening.

Water temperature: 50°F–60°F.

Duration: Several seconds to 10 minutes. Do this twice a day, morning and late afternoon.

Warning: Treading is addictive!

Note: Cold toe and footbaths should not be used if the following conditions exist: rheumatism of toes and ankles, sciatica, neuralgia of the bladder, pelvic inflammation, irritable bladder or rectum.

COLD SHALLOW TOE BATH
(short)

THERAPEUTIC USES

Create intense reaction in pelvic area	Decongest lungs
	Decongest head

Method

Add ice cubes to a small amount of cold water in the bathtub, or in a large dishpan. Dip in the toes for 30 seconds. Rub entire foot vigorously. Return toes to bath, and keep repeating the action until the feet become red. End the treatment by rubbing the feet dry. Rapidly tap the sole of the foot.

COLD RUNNING WATER FOOT BATH
(short)

THERAPEUTIC USES

Insomnia	General fatigue
Congestion in head	Moderate depression

Method

Sit on the edge of the bathtub and place your feet and ankles under cold running tap water for several seconds to several minutes depending on your tolerance for cold.

PROLONGED COLD FOOT BATH

THERAPEUTIC USES

Sprains   Inflamed bunions

Method

First, warm the feet under pleasantly hot water. Run moderately cold water into the tub, and soak feet to just below the ankles, or if working on ankle sprain, above the ankles. (See also Alternate Hot and Cold Foot Bath for sprain.)

Water temperature: 60°F–70°F.

Duration: About 10 minutes.

Do not use during menstruation, bladder infection, or if there is any inflammation of the chest, abdomen, or pelvic organs.

WARM FOOT BATH
(short)

THERAPEUTIC USES

When vigorous cold   For soreness of the neck
    foot baths cannot be used   For circulation problems
As preparation for cold   To overcome congestion in
    foot baths   other parts of the body

The warm temperature foot bath is more comfortable for the very young, the very weak, and the very old. It should *not* be used by those whose feet perspire profusely.

Method

Run warm water from the tap into the tub and soak the feet for several minutes.

Water temperature: 80°F–92°F.

To achieve a temperature of 85°F, use one quart of boiling water to four quarts of cold water. To achieve a temperature of 92°F, use one quart of boiling water to three quarts of cold water.

HOT FOOT BATH
(short and prolonged)

THERAPEUTIC USES

Relieve cramps in feet and leg   Overcome insomnia
Relieve pain of gout   Prepare body for any hot
Relieve menstrual cramps   water therapy
Relieve neuralgic pains   Relieve sore throat or cold

Hot foot baths are an excellent water therapy for drawing blood from inflamed parts of the body, or drawing congestion away from an organ. Hot foot baths will speed up the body's reaction to a salt massage bath or a shallow (sit or hip) bath.

Method

Use a large dishpan or the bathtub. Start with warm water and increase the heat until it is as hot as you can tolerate. If you have no bath thermometer, use 1 quart of boiling water to 2 quarts of cold water to produce a hot bath at 106°F. Or 2 quarts of boiling water and 4 quarts of cold water for a gallon and a half at 106°F. If the water gets cool, withdraw one cup of water and replace with two cups of boiling water.

Renew *cold compress to forehead* every several minutes to prevent head congestion.

End every hot treatment with a lukewarm, then cool, sponging or shower directed to the soles of the feet. Wrap the feet in a towel and dry carefully. Keep them wrapped for about 15 minutes.

When the hot foot bath is used to relieve a sore throat or to abort a cold, add 1 tablespoon mustard powder to 1 quart of hot water, and add this mixture to the foot bath.

When the hot foot bath is in preparation for perspiration-inducing water therapies, add hayflower extract or strong hayflower tea or oatstraw tea. Or add a tablespoon of a stimulating herb powder, such as mustard, or ⅛ teaspoon of powdered cayenne pepper, or ½ teaspoon of powdered ginger or strong rosemary tea or rosemary extract. Dissolve any ingredient in hot water *before* adding to the foot bath. Use only hayflower or oatstraw if there are open sores or broken skin.

Temperature: 106°F–115°F.

Duration: 10–30 minutes, depending on the case and tolerance to heat.

HOT AND COLD CONTRAST FOOT BATH

Hot Water: 100°F–110°F	Cold Water: 40°F–55°F
1: 3 minutes	2: 1 minute
3: 3 minutes	4: 1 minute
5: 3 minutes	6: 1 minute
7: 3 minutes	8: 1 minute
9: 3 minutes	

ALTERNATE HOT AND COLD FOOT BATH

THERAPEUTIC USES

Toothache	Passive swelling of the
Neuralgia	ankles
Headache (use cold compress	Foot infections
on head)	Chilblains
Catarrh	Blood poisoning

Congestion of abdomen   To warm up the body for
Congestion of pelvic organs   other treatments
Cold body   In addition to some
Cold feet   other water therapies

An alternate hot and cold foot bath is a very useful water therapy because the heat sedates, and the cold stimulates the feet and other parts of the body connected by reflex to the feet. This alternate bath is frequently used in treating sprained ankles.

Method

Use two containers. Fill one with hot water (100°F–110°F), the other with cold tap water (about 60°F). Steep both feet up to the ankles in the hot water for 3 minutes. Withdraw and plunge the feet into the container of cold water for 20–30 seconds. Repeat the process 3 times. End with cold water. Carefully wipe the feet dry.

The beneficial effect of this bath lasts quite a long time.

ALTERNATE HOT AND COLD LEG BATH

THERAPEUTIC USES

Insomnia   Suppressed menstruation
Pulmonary congestion   Ovarian congestion
Painful period   Pelvic pain

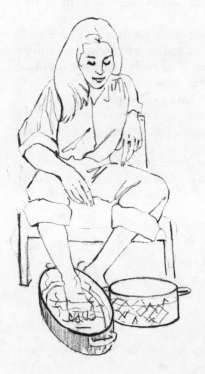

ALTERNATE HOT AND COLD FOOT BATH

Fig. 14. Any alternate hot and cold application of water alternately sedates and stimulates the body. Such a foot bath has a profound effect, especially since many of the nerves and reflex points connected to other organs are found in the feet.

This foot bath is used in rehabilitation of many foot injuries since it creates new circulation patterns. The alternate hot and cold foot bath is also effective in relieving congestion in many other organs, and is helpful in headaches, some ankle swelling, foot infections, and chilblains (minor frostbite).

Steep one or both feet in hot water for 3 minutes, then plunge immediately into the cold water for 20–30 seconds. Repeat 3 times. Unless specifically noted, end all such foot baths with cold water.

Method

Follow the same procedure as for the Alternate Hot and Cold Foot Bath (above), but plunge feet into the water up to the *calves.* Keep feet in the hot bath for 2 minutes; in the cold bath for 20 seconds. Repeat 6 times.

Do not use this bath if cystitis (bladder infection) or any congestion of the prostate, uterus, or kidney is present.

HAYFLOWER FOOT BATHS

THERAPEUTIC USES

Heal open cuts on feet

Reduce inflammation of nail bed on toe

Control profuse sweating of feet

Overcome discomfort of tight shoes

Reduce hematoma (tissue filled with blood)

Hayflower foot baths are a wonderful remedy for certain foot problems, and they also can be used to induce detoxification in other areas of the body. (See Chapters 7 and 10.)

Method

Make a strong hayflower tea by pouring a quart of boiling water over 1–2 handfuls of dried hayflower blossoms. Steep for 15–25 minutes (the longer the better), strain, and when cold add to the foot bath of your choice.

The temperature of most hayflower foot baths should be tepid (about 85°F). The baths may last from a few minutes to about 15 minutes, or slightly longer, depending on comfort. End each hayflower foot bath with a cold sponging, and vigorous towel drying.

For *swollen feet* use a short cold foot bath (a few minutes), or a swift cold jet shower to the feet, and then apply hayflower compresses. The herb helps the pores of the skin to open and thus encourages a discharge of internally stored toxins.

Hayflower is available in extract form from Bio-Kosma, a Swiss firm. It is distributed in the United States by Weleda. Dried hayflower is available from local or mail order suppliers. (See Resources, page 232.)

OATSTRAW FOOT BATHS

THERAPEUTIC USES

Sore feet	Foot blisters
Knots on feet	Pain of chronic gout, arthritis,
Sores that develop pus	rheumatism
Ingrown toe nails	

Method

Pour a handful or two of oatstraw (depending on strength of preparation desired), into a quart of boiling water and simmer for 20–30 minutes. Steep for 30 minutes or so, strain, and when cold add to a hot foot bath to create a *tepid* foot bath. Sponge feet with cold water, and dry with coarse towel.

Oatstraw is a *very* strong detoxifier. Repeat this procedure only three times a week, 15 minutes at a time, until the condition clears up. Repeat only twice a week for persons in a weakened condition.

(10)

Hand Baths

Partial hand baths act directly on the hands and work by reflex action on other areas of the body. Like foot baths they can have a profound effect in alleviating any number of ailments. See page 16 for reflex areas.

COLD HAND BATHS

THERAPEUTIC USES

Control excessive perspiration of hands

Check nose bleed

Lower temperature in ear inflammation

Relieve sunstroke or overheating

Ice held in the hand or hands will check a nose bleed. To prevent future nose bleeds, frequently immerse hands in cold water of 45°F–60°F, 3–5 minutes at a time. Dry hands with a coarse towel.

Excessive perspiration of the hands can also be controlled by frequent cold water hand baths, as above.

Cold water baths can be used both to lower the temperature of the external auditory ear canal, and to lessen the pressure of the arteries in the brain

Whenever there is a wound or inflammation on the arms or hands, dip the hands up to the elbow in cold hayflower water. To do this, add a tablespoon of hayflower bath extract (Bio-Kosma) to a quart of tepid water and cool, or, alternatively, steep a handful of dried hayflower blossoms in a quart of boiling water for 20–30 minutes (the longer the better).

Then let the water cool. It is not necessary to strain out the flowers. Keep the hand or arm immersed in the bath for 15 minutes. Dry well afterward.

HOT HAND BATH

THERAPEUTIC USES

Chronic skin diseases	Writer's cramp
Local inflammations	Telegrapher's cramp
Asthma	Needleperson's cramp
Emphysema	In preparation for cold water
Abscess of nail tip	therapy such as cold half
Inflammation of nail tip	bath or cold shower
Tennis player's wrist	

For most of the above problems, soak hands in hot water for several seconds to several minutes, depending on your tolerance. Repeat 3–4 times a day, or as often as needed. While your hands are soaking, move your fingers to increase circulation. Cool the hands briefly with a cold water splash, and dry carefully.

Chronic asthma attacks may be alleviated by plunging hands and forearms in very hot water for several seconds. Repeat 3–4 times a day. Follow each hot immersion with a brief cold splash or sponging, and dry the hands.

An inflammation that occurs at the nail bed and which causes pus is called a felon. Felons are terribly painful. Both the inflammation and pain will be reduced by immersing the arm up to the elbow in hot water for 10 seconds several times a day. Hayflower extract or strong hayflower tea can be added to this water to increase the anti-inflammation effect.

ALTERNATE HOT AND COLD HAND BATH

THERAPEUTIC USES

As general tonic to improve circulation of wrists and hands
After treatment for fracture
After treatment for wrist sprains
To help control mild hemorrhages in other parts of the body
To help relieve minor frostbite (chilblains)
For cold hands

Have two containers: one with extremely hot water (as hot as you can tolerate), and one with very cold water.

Plunge hands in hot water for 3 minutes. Withdraw, and plunge the hands into cold water for ½ minute. Repeat 3 times. Always end this alternate bath with *cold water* in order to restore muscle and internal tone.

For very cold hands, start with a cold water rub, then alternate between the hot and cold immersions.

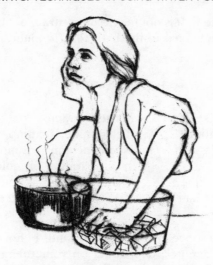

ALTERNATE HOT AND COLD HAND BATH

Fig. 15.   There are many reflex points in the hand. Thus hand or arm baths can affect other parts of the body, and sometimes alter a disease state in the entire system.

A cold hand bath checks a nose bleed, and a hot bath relieves many athletic or overuse problems of the hand, and is a useful tool in alleviating asthma attacks.

Alternate hot and cold hand baths help restore healthy circulation to the wrists and hands, and should also be used in most injury rehabilitation of this area. Use hot water for 3 minutes, and then cold water for ½ minute. Repeat several times. Always end with a cold water plunge.

(11)

Herb and Medicated Baths

There are many herb and pharmaceutical substances that can be added to baths to produce special effects.

Water by itself has a remarkable, almost magic ability to alter the body state. Depending on the specific need, water will decrease or increase muscle tone, reduce pain, or generate energy. The addition of certain herbal and pharmaceutical substances to the water is a twin present to the body. Some herbs soothe, others sedate or stimulate, and others soften the skin. Most important is the ability of some substances to hasten perspiration, to stimulate release of stored toxins from within the body. This ability helps to overcome many acute attacks, and can improve a chronic condition.

All of the following substances are excellent, and some have overlapping effects. I suggest you try each of them at various times in order to note your personal reaction. Then, if you need any of these substances in an emergency, you will know which work the most effectively for you.

Oatmeal — excellent for skin problems

Salt — large amounts of salt added to the bath water help heal and tranquilize; a *salt rub* is cheap and quickly invigorates the skin before any kind of bath

Apple cider vinegar — combats fatigue and restores the body's natural acid covering

Sage — helps stimulate the sweat glands when added to bath water

Nutmeg — can increase perspiration when added to bath water; also said to be helpful in radiation detoxification

Rosemary — stimulates and increases the circulation of the blood

Pine — helps to open the pores, soften and stimulate the skin, and cure skin rashes

Hayflower and **oatstraw** — immediately releases skin impurities

Bran — softens the skin

Fennel and **nettle** — mild detoxifiers

Epsom salts — a strong perspiration-inducer and muscle relaxer, *but it may be too strong for persons in a weakened state*

Ginger powder tea and ginger root tea — relax sore muscles, tone the skin, and greatly improve sluggish circulation; ginger is so stimulating that it must be used only in small amounts at first, and then gradually increased to your tolerance

Sulphur — a general healing aid; also helps certain skin problems

Borax, starch, and **bicarbonate of soda** — general skin aids

Dead Sea salts — helps restore body functions after injury

Vitabath and **Algemarin** — excellent skin softeners, relaxers, and general body toners

All of the above are inexpensive and easy to use. The various herbs can be obtained from local health food stores, or by mail from botanical suppliers. Vitabath, Algemarin, pine extract, Dead Sea salts, sulphur, and Aveeno (colloidal oatmeal) are available in drugstores and some department stores.

Never buy too large a quantity of herbs in advance, as they lose their potency in about a year. You can make strong tinctures or extracts of any herb yourself. (For directions, see my book *The Complete Herbal Guide to Natural Health and Beauty.*) These will last a very long time, and you can add small amounts of the tincture or extract to the bathwater or compress as needed.

APPLE CIDER VINEGAR BATH

THERAPEUTIC USES

Overcome fatigue	Relieve poison ivy
Detoxify	Relieve sun burn
Relieve itchiness	Cosmetic for the skin

Apple cider vinegar is a reliable, inexpensive bath aid. I purchase it in quantity so that I never run out and usually transfer the vinegar to decorative flasks and keep one in each bathroom. I add about one cup to my bath. But if I am trying to overcome fatigue, I first pour a little of the apple cider vinegar into the cup of my hand, and splash it over my shoulders, arms, back, and chest. I then slide into the warm to hot bath and soak with my entire body submerged. Next, I let out the warm water and slowly replace it with cold water which I splash first over my feet, and then sponge over my entire body, allowing it to dribble down my spine. This cold water splash never fails to invigorate and restore energy.

Add 2 cups of apple cider vinegar to the bathwater to overcome itchiness or relieve poison ivy attacks.

SALT MASSAGE BATH

THERAPEUTIC USES

To abort an oncoming cold	Relieve rheumatism/gout
Restore circulation	Add buoyancy
Overcome sluggishness	Eliminate dead skin

This is a must when you are feeling low. The salt friction on the body, along with other tonic therapies and relaxing warm baths (filled with herbal substances or coarse salt as described throughout this section), can actually keep you going through stress periods. I always keep a decorative jar of salt on a shelf near my bath so I can make up a quick salt paste for the massage.

Plain coarse salt or sea salt can be used in two different ways, or combined into a consecutive treatment. When massaged, as a paste, over unbroken skin, salt acts as a body stimulant, increases the circulation in anemic conditions, helps to overcome mild depressions, increases the

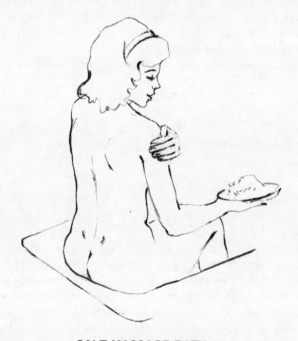

SALT MASSAGE BATH

Fig. 16. Feeling tired, or on the brink of a cold? Try a reenergizing salt-paste friction rub. The salt massage increases internal circulation, helps overcome fatigue, creates a feeling of well-being, and eliminates dead skin.

After this massage, soak in a light-to-heavy salt solution bath, or add apple cider vinegar, pine essence, or any of a dozen effective herbal solutions to soak away fatigue or anxiety. End the bath with a cold water splash and a vigorous terry towel rub.

tone of the body before or after an infection, and can help to overcome the body trauma caused by excessive drinking. This massage may be used separately, or in combination with an immersion salt bath.

Massage

A vigorous massage with a slushy paste of salt and warm water increases circulation; cleanses the skin and therefore intensifies elimination through the skin; stimulates both the sebaceous glands and the nervous system. The massage acts as a tonic on the blood vessels and other tissues of the body. The total feeling after this rub is one of rejuvenation and renewed vitality.

Sit nude on the edge of a bathtub filled with warm water. Pour a handful of salt into an unbreakable container or the cup of your hand. Add small amounts of water until you have a thick paste. Apply the salt paste in slow, circular motions over the body from the shoulders to the feet. This salt massage may also be applied while you are sitting with both feet in hot water. In this case, also apply a damp cold compress to the forehead.

After the massage, either wash off the salt with a gentle or jet shower, or a cold sponging, or slide into the bath which has meanwhile been filled with moderately warm to hot water. Soak the entire body. The massage should only take a few minutes.

Do not use a salt massage if skin lesions or inflammation is present.

SALT BATH

THERAPEUTIC USES

To relax	After too much sitting
To release tension	For sluggish skin
For menopause	

Coarse salt can be added to any bath to produce buoyancy, and additional salt may be massaged on the back during the bath. The more salt there is in the water, the greater will be the feeling of relaxation and refreshment.

I find such salt baths, even with only a cup or two of salt, very calming for the body, totally relaxing, and almost hypnotic. The greater the amount of salt, the more the perspiration. Small amounts such as a cup do not increase the perspiration. As little as 5 pounds of common coarse salt will approximate natural sea water which is between 1% and 7% salt. This acts as a mild tonic on the body in the same way that bathing in the sea creates a feeling of mild euphoria.

I use the combined salt massage and salt bath to overcome sluggishness from sitting at the typewriter most of the day. It is also one of my many weapons to help abort an incipient cold.

Take long salt baths in *tepid* water whenever possible as the salt holds the heat very well. When a tonic effect is desired, use colder water (75°F–65°F) and immerse the body for 1–2 minutes. End the bath with a cool sponging or a needle shower.

This bath is useful for women in menopause, and for those who need to increase skin activity, but whose weakness or cardiac condition do not allow stronger baths.

"Algemarin" is a sea-algae vitamin foam-bath available in many department stores. It tones, freshens, and revitalizes the body. Dead Sea salts, available in health food stores, also have restorative and softening powers. Both are excellent bath products.

OATMEAL BATH

THERAPEUTIC USES
> Soothe the skin
> Overcome itchiness
> Overcome hives
> Relieve sunburn, chafing, windburn, dishpan hands

Oatmeal is one of the most extraordinary herbs. It is not only useful and dependable in soothing and nourishing the body internally, it also coats, soothes, and restores rough skin. It is a must for baby bathwater as it overcomes the acidity of urine or diaper rash. It can also be used both as a paste on the body before the bath and in the bathwater to relieve the most stubborn chafing welts between the legs.

Method

To use oatmeal in the bath, either blend raw oatmeal into tiny particles or use a prepared, colloidal, suspended oatmeal. Add up to one cup oatmeal to tepid or warm bathwater.

Oatmeal in the bathwater mollifies windburn and sunburn, and relieves itchiness. For treating poison ivy attacks, I alternate between using oatmeal baths with Aveeno (the prepared, colloidal, suspended particles of oatmeal, obtained in the drugstore), and apple cider vinegar baths. While I prefer using Aveeno, it is quite expensive. You can prepare your own oatmeal body-soother by blending the rough cooking oatmeal into a powder. Do this in advance, bottle and label, and keep in the medicine chest.

HAYFLOWER BATH

THERAPEUTIC USES
> Detoxify

Hayflower—the very word connotes vast fields of newly grown grass. When I was a child, my family and I collected these flowers, dried them on a huge screen, and stored them in brown paper bags. Sometimes we sewed the hayflowers into minihandkerchief pouches. These we plunged into a quart of boiling water, and we then poured the extracted "tea" from these pouches into the bathwater whenever we wanted to ease muscular tension, or, especially, to extract toxins before a cold or during an acute bacterial attack. Healthy persons may use this potent extractor as often as they please, *but weak or ill persons are advised to use these flowers in moderation.* Once a week is often enough for chronic rheumatism, or other chronic health problems. See the specific listings in Part III for details.

Method

Make a strong tea of the dried hayflowers with about 3 cups of the flowers to 2 quarts of boiling water. Pour the boiling water over the flowers, steep for 15–30 minutes and strain. Add this strained liquid to any partial or full bath. Add tepid, warm, or hot water, depending on the amount of perspiration you wish to induce.

There is an excellent Swiss Alpine Hayflower Bath Extract available through Weleda, South Main Street, Spring Valley, New York. This is excellent in helping to abort a cold and in overcoming the effects of a poisoned insect bite.

Other Water Therapy Uses

Hayflower *compresses,* or hayflower *dipped shirts,* placed on children will act quickly to bring out the internal eruptions in many children's diseases. See the specific listings in Part III.

Hayflower *arm baths* are excellent for any inflammation or wounds on the arms and fingers.

Hayflower *foot baths* will help reduce inflammation and pus in the nail bed of the toes, and relieve swelling around open cuts, or tissues filled with blood after an injury. They also help with the problem of sweating feet and they have a remarkable effect on swollen feet.

Picking Hayflowers

Hayflowers are frequently the yellow, sweet-scented vernal grass. But this is the very same grass that gives so much trouble to hay fever victims. You can make a tincture of these hayflowers by soaking them in brandy. A sniff or two in each nostril during a hay fever attack will usually produce instantaneous relief.

Another excellent detoxifying hayflower is the aromatic clivers, sometimes called goosegrass.

OATSTRAW BATH

THERAPEUTIC USES

Detoxify	Knots on feet
Diseases of the bladder	Sores that turn to pus
Ingrown toenails	Pain of arthritis, gout,
Blisters on the feet	rheumatism
Sore feet	

The straw left over when oat is harvested is a very important detoxifying substance. It can be used alone or in combination with hayflower.

The chemicals in hayflowers can be released by steeping in boiling water, but oatstraw must be simmered for 20 minutes or more. Then, steep, strain, and pour into tepid or warm temperature bathwater.

End each bath with a cold sponging, and vigorous friction towel rub.

Bladder Problems

For bladder problems take one 10-minute *warm* oatstraw bath a month. After a month, plan a series of *cold* oatstraw baths for several months. Then take the warm baths in the same sequence until the problems are eliminated.

Note: The action of the oatstraw is so strong that it may be debilitating for weak persons.

Foot Problems

Use footsoaks with oatstraw for sore feet, knots on the feet, sores that develop pus, ingrown toenails, and blisters on the feet. Such baths are also useful for the pain of chronic gout, arthritis, and rheumatism.

CHAMOMILE BATH

THERAPEUTIC USES

To soothe skin	To open pores and eliminate
As antiseptic	blackheads
For digestive problems	As sleeping aid

The mild apple-smelling herb chamomile is one of the most versatile of herbs.

Method

Pour a pint of boiling water over a handful of chamomile flowers in a nonaluminum container, steep for 15 minutes, strain, and pour the strained liquid into a steamy hot bath. Relax in the bath for about 10 minutes. This will open the pores of the body and the face. However, the hot bath will cause lassitude and deplete muscle tone, so end this bath by splashing cold water on your *body* to restore the tone. Do *not* use cold water on your face, but as quickly as possible get out of the bath and gently push out facial blackheads with two cotton swabs. (See instructions for chamomile facials on page 60.)

Chamomile helps relieve internal digestive spasms. Add it to the bathwater as above, or pour it on a large, natural sponge and gently massage the abdomen in clockwise, rotating motions. See also the listing of specific problems in Part III.

PINE BATH

THERAPEUTIC USES

Recover after vigorous exercise	Relax, especially if
Relieve breathing problems in	excessively nervous
asthma, bronchitis	Increased skin action
Overcome fatigue	Eliminate blackheads
Increase perspiration	

The delightful and heady aroma of pine is available in extract form in several effective products. My favorites are the liquid and/or the condensed "tablet" products from the Black Forest of Germany.

Those of you who have had the pleasure of walking through a pine forest will undoubtedly recall the sensation of being able to breathe deeper and lighter. Pine has that kind of effect on the lungs. This in turn gives the kidneys a boost, and they function better.

Method

If the bath is intended to relieve fatigue after exercise, or to relax, fill the bathtub with water slightly lower than body temperature, 95°F–97°F—and pour in one capful of the pine extract. Immerse your entire body. Remain in the bath for 15–30 minutes.

If you want to produce sweating, start the bath at the above temperature, add the pine, and increase the hot water to 102°F. Remain in the bath for 10 minutes.

If breathing difficulties are the main focus of the bath, take only a partial sit bath. Sit on a rubber pillow that is placed on the side of the tub. Wear a towel or a shirt on your torso. Use tepid water, and get out of the bath as soon as breathing difficulties are somewhat eased.

In an emergency, if no pine extract is available, you can add 4 ounces of turpentine (a pine product) to the water to aid the breathing activities. *However, when using turpentine it is imperative that you keep the genital area out of the bath water. Do not use turpentine if there are any open sores on the lower part of the body, as the turpentine may irritate the skin.*

A small tablet of the concentrated pine extract, or a dollop of the green liquified pine added to warm water in the bath, reddens the surface of the skin. When blood is drawn to the surface in this type of action, it increases the number of red and white blood cells. Pine also has a special action on the substance, cholestrine, which accumulates in the pores of the skin. It is therefore helpful in controlling blackheads.

Pine will increase the tendency of the body to perspire. Run hot water in the bath and add the pine extract according to directions on the bottle or tablet box. The aroma will make the bath feel luxurious, and the pine will relieve muscle fatigue, help in quickly eliminating debris developed during athletic activity, and aid in perspiration (this is especially useful if you are catching a cold).

BRAN BATH

THERAPEUTIC USES

Relieve itching	Invigorate and tone skin and nerves
Clean surface of skin	Alleviate nervous conditions

Bran is the outer covering of wheat, and is an essential fiber in preventing and overcoming constipation. Bran can be prepared separately and strained before placing in the bathwater, or zipped into close mesh pouches. It makes the water milky white.

Bran has also been used for thousands of years for various skin conditions, and will help with any generalized itching or dermatitis. It softens the skin, and leaves a coating of fine particles on the skin. It can soothe any irritation of the skin. It also subtly eliminates dead skin cells and rough scales.

Bran in the bathwater is useful for nervous conditions since it helps to invigorate the body and tone up the skin and the nerves at the same time.

Bran can be added to several alkaline substances, such as sodium bicarbonate and borax for antiseptic purposes, and starch for cooling the skin and allaying itching, chafing, poison ivy, and eczema.

Method

Sew several handfuls of bran into a cheesecloth pouch. Soak in very *hot* water for several minutes. Fill the bathtub with neutral water—slightly under body temperature (96°F). Place the pouch in the water and squeeze it until the water turns milky white.

Another method is slightly messier, but has a wonderful effect on certain dermatological problems. Close the filter of the bathtub with the bran cheesecloth pouch and fill the bathtub with warm water. Get in. While the bath is filling, sponge your body with hot water. Remove the cheesecloth, put a stopper on the filter, and rub your body with the cheesecloth. The bran friction rub invigorates and soothes.

Always finish a bran bath with vigorous towel rub of the body. If you can, allow the fine particles of bran to stay *on* the body. If you prefer, you may sponge them off with tepid or cool water.

Water temperature: 95°F–98°F.

Duration: bran baths can last from a half hour up to several hours, if desired.

CORNSTARCH, BORAX, SODIUM BICARBONATE BATHS

THERAPEUTIC USES

To soothe skin

As antiseptic

Several household products can be added to the bath. Cornstarch is an excellent dusting powder that absorbs excess perspiration, and, when added to the bath, it is also an effective cooling agent. Used alone, or with bran or oatmeal, it moderates the itchiness of poison ivy, poison oak, eczema, and prickly heat. Add between a cup and a pound of the cornstarch to a warm bath.

Borax is an antiseptic that makes the bathwater soft and slippery and the body feel very pleasant. It tends to be slightly drying, however. For full effect, add between one-half to one cup to warm bathwater.

The 1887 United States Dispensatory notes that some physicians were successful in treating ringworm of the scalp with a borax-vinegar wash. This consisted of a large pinch of borax plus 2 ounces of distilled vinegar. Combine the items in larger proportions for a bath for ringworm patients.

Sodium bicarbonate in the bathwater opens the pores, cleanses the body, acts as a mild antiseptic, and relieves itching and skin irritation. Use from half a pound to a pound in neutral temperature water.

EPSOM SALT BATH

THERAPEUTIC USES

Increase perspiration	Relieve neuritis, lumbago, arthritis,
Abort an illness	sciatica, rheumatism
Eliminate toxic debris	Relieve muscular fatigue
Help control catarrh	

Epsom salts added to hot bathwater will induce profuse perspiration, and this bath should be used particularly before the onset of a cold, flu, or other infection. Such baths are also helpful in relaxing the body after strenuous exercise, and for pain relief in chronic arthritis, sciatica, and rheumatism. However, these baths tend also to deplete the body, *so do not take them if you are weak or have heart trouble, arteriosclerosis, diabetes, or are postoperative.* Also, epsom salts are very potent and may bother some people.

Method

Put protective material such as a rubber sheet or an old wool blanket on the bed.

Fill the tub with hot water to your utmost temperature tolerance. Dissolve from one cup to one pound of the epsom salts. The more salts, the more perspiration. Before entering the tub, apply the first of several consecutive large cold compresses to forehead and head, and then sit submerged in the hot water for 10–20 minutes. While in the tub, drink a hot herbal tea—peppermint, thyme, sage, etc.—or some other fluid to further increase perspiration and replace lost fluids.

The length of time you stay in the bath depends on your age and health, but since the heat and the perspiration tend to be weakening, no matter what age you are, get out of the bath slowly.

Do not dry, but cover your body with large towels and go to bed immediately. Lie under a coverlet, and allow body perspiration to continue. If you fall asleep at this time, wait until morning to sponge off with tepid water. Conclude the wash with a cool water sponging and a vigorous rub to dry the body. If you do not fall asleep after a half an hour or so, sponge off as above and dry vigorously. Then, change bedclothes, go back to bed, and enjoy a long, restful sleep.

SULPHUR BATH

THERAPEUTIC USES

Relieve skin ailments   Relieve pain in arthritis, chronic
Heal the body   gout, neuritis
Mild antiseptic   Overcome acne
Mild antiparasite

Natural sulphur waters have helped patients to overcome a wide variety of skin ailments, and to heal the body internally as well as externally.

Method

Fill the bathtub with tepid water and add from half a cup to a cup and a half of colloidal (fine suspended particles) sulphur, or sulphur-bath preparation. Sit submerged in the bath for 10–20 minutes. The sulphur is reduced chemically to sulphurated hydrogen, and, when absorbed by the skin, has a great healing, cleansing, and antiseptic effect.

Sulphur baths are also helpful with acne.

Bath temperature: 95°F–102°F.

ASCORBIC ACID BATH

THERAPEUTIC USES

Allergy attack   Hemorrhoids
Infection

I would never have thought of using ascorbic acid powder (vitamin C), in the bath, except that on a hunch I poured 3 tablespoons in a warm bath during a sudden allergy attack. Shortly after this, to my amazement, the sneezing stopped altogether!

Dr. John Hanks, an athletic consultant for the Denver Broncos and Denver Nuggets, who is also a proponent of water therapy, recommends using ascorbic acid sit baths (shallow baths) to treat hemorrhoids. Hemorrhoids are a problem that afflict many athletes and dancers, and Dr. Hanks feels that the addition of ascorbic acid to the bath greatly speeds up the healing process. Add 1 cup of the powder to 5 quarts of cool water (the water should be as cool as you can tolerate). Sit in the bath for 3–15 minutes, depending on your tolerance.

SHAMPOO

THERAPEUTIC USES

Clean hair   Increase skin action
Clean scalp   Overcome energy blocks
Clean body   Stimulate acupuncture pressure points
Detoxify

Did you ever stop to think why you feel so good after you take a cleansing bath and shampoo your hair? Shampooing with water, a good emollient, nondetergent soap, and hand pressure or friction materials, not only cleanses and refreshes the body, but eliminates dead skin cells, and opens the pores of the skin. This in turn helps to pass unneeded material out of the system. A shampoo also stimulates the internal organs —acting like an electric light switch in "turning on" crucial hand, foot, face, and scalp pressure points. This is why a strong hair wash and scalp rub (with careful drying) can sometimes turn the tide in eliminating a head cold.

When you shampoo, the protective acid mantle of the skin is gradually washed away. It is necessary to restore this acid barrier. I do this by using diluted apple cider vinegar as one of my restorative hair rinses.

There are many excellent herbal shampoos and soaps on the market. Many are made from pure products which will heal the body, tone up the skin, soften the skin, and also restore the pH balance. In addition to the excellent products found in most health food stores today, the following are some of my favorite mail order firms: Caswell Massey has a truly international selection of interesting shampoos and soaps. The Weleda Company manufactures and imports Swiss and German bath products, including a great chestnut shampoo which is useful if you have hard water. "Culpeper The Herbalist" is a series of stores in Great Britain, started by the Society of Herbalists, that sell very high quality shampoos and soaps (I like the cucumber and almond oil products). Another unusual mail order source is D. Napier's and Sons of Edinburgh. This organization of family herbalists opened its doors in 1860 and manufactures a very healing, emollient slippery elm soap. See Resource List.

Shampoo for Hair

You should choose a shampoo and rinse that suit your hair texture and will restore your pH balance. Dry, normal, and oily hair all need a different shampoo and rinse. It therefore pays to experiment with the different natural-based shampoos on the market. Do not use a regular cake soap as a shampoo—it will dull the hair. And be wary of the highly promoted anti-dandruff shampoos. They contain chemicals which can sometimes irritate. In general, proper scalp stimulation, frequent brushing, cleansing with a mild shampoo, and taking appropriate amounts of vitamins, exercise, rest, and sunshine will make the skin and hair lustrous and healthy.

If you have a chronic disease condition, you should wash your hair and scalp frequently in order to stimulate circulation and eliminate toxins from the body.

Shampoo for Body

If you go to a spa or an old-fashioned Turkish Bath you will be lathered from head to toe with soap, and a skilled practioner will scrub your body with a large scrubbing brush. The scrubbing stimulates your body so that you will feel tingly and wide awake. After the scrub you will shower—always ending with cold water. Then, you will be encouraged to take a short nap. Because of the exhilarating scrub, you will fall asleep instantly and awaken totally refreshed.

This body shampoo can be somewhat duplicated at home. Begin by soaking the body in a vegetable oil (olive oil is preferred). Soak in a bathtub full of warm to hot water. Soap the body completely with a natural, non-detergent, hard milled soap, and scrub with a loofah, an aloes brush, a natural bristle brush, or a hand crocheted Israeli or Mexican hemp washcloth. Scrub gently at first, then work up to a vigorous scrubbing. If the skin is very delicate or sensitive, use a large natural sponge for the first few weeks and then graduate to the friction mitt or brush.

Other shampoos may be preceded with a salt massage to increase circulation.

End each bath with cool to cold water, especially on the feet. Splash apple cider vinegar, or diluted apple cider vinegar and rose water over the body. For a truly exhilarating feeling, use the Scots shower—alternate long hot and short cold streams. Vigorously rub the body dry.

See also pages 129–131 for additional information on detoxification bath/shampoo techniques for chronic diseases.

(12)

Packs

Packs are an ancient concept. Water and cloths have long been used to create and to develop specific states in the body. Each step of these procedures should be used cautiously. Test and check each step to ensure personal safety.

DAMP COLD SHEET PACK
(or Cold Double Body Compress)

THERAPEUTIC USES

Fever	Muscular problems
Children's diseases	Menopause heat
Nervousness	As tonic
Oncoming cold or flu	As sedative
Skin diseases	As elimatative
Joint problems	

This pack is the *most effective and powerful* of all the water therapies.

While the directions for this pack may seem complicated at first, it is actually only a long, double body compress in which the legs are separated by a layer of cloth. This pack is exceptional in helping to overcome fevers, and a three-quarter or half pack may be used several times a day. It is also very helpful for most chronic diseases, in detoxifying the body, and for aborting an oncoming flu or cold attack.

The action of this compress or body pack is like that of a giant detoxifying magnet. For this reason, except in the case of fever, do not use it too often. Do not use this technique after meals. (See "Cold Double Compress" section for three-quarter and half trunk or smaller packs.)

Method

1. Prepare a hot water bottle. Prepare the bed with protective material by laying 2 large blankets so that the ends are lower than the sides of the bed. Then place a large, dry white sheet on top of the blankets. You will later lay cold wet sheet on top of the dry sheet. See item #4. The hot water bottle will warm the feet.

2. Have a perspiration-inducing drink, such as peppermint, hayflower, or oatstraw tea, ready at the bedside, and by the bath.

3. Have containers of cold water for the cold compress at bath and bedside.

4. Prepare the damp wet sheet by plunging a large white cotton cloth or sheet into cold water, and wringing it out so that it is damp, but not too wet. Keep it in the sink, to either apply it directly after the bath while you are standing, or place it on the bed on the dry sheet for when you emerge from the bath.

5. Prepare a full hot bath, or a hot foot bath. A full hot bath is

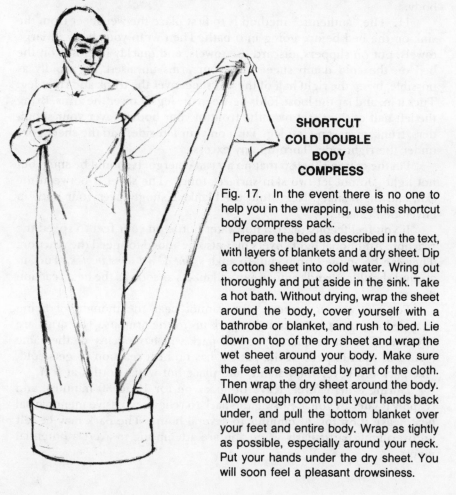

**SHORTCUT
COLD DOUBLE
BODY
COMPRESS**

Fig. 17. In the event there is no one to help you in the wrapping, use this shortcut body compress pack.

Prepare the bed as described in the text, with layers of blankets and a dry sheet. Dip a cotton sheet into cold water. Wring out thoroughly and put aside in the sink. Take a hot bath. Without drying, wrap the sheet around the body, cover yourself with a bathrobe or blanket, and rush to bed. Lie down on top of the dry sheet and wrap the wet sheet around your body. Make sure the feet are separated by part of the cloth. Then wrap the dry sheet around the body. Allow enough room to put your hands back under, and pull the bottom blanket over your feet and entire body. Wrap as tightly as possible, especially around your neck. Put your hands under the dry sheet. You will soon feel a pleasant drowsiness.

preferred for total relaxation, sedation, and perspiration induction. You can increase the detoxification effect by adding up to 5 cups of epsom salts, a cup of pine extract, a cup of hayflower tea, or a tablespoon of hayflower extract to the bathwater.

6. Void bladder.

7. If you are trying to abort a cold or the flu, consider also taking a cold water enema before the bath.

8. Apply a cold compress to the forehead. Enter the hot bath, or take a hot foot bath (see pages 65–66). Drink herbal drinks. The bath may last from 15 to 30 minutes depending on your comfort and vitality. (Hot baths tend to sap the energy from the body.) Perspiration starts.

9. Get out of the bath.

10. There are two methods of wrapping. The short cut is to lift your hands, and wrap the cold damp sheet around your body. Wrap some towels around your body, go to the bed, discard the towels and lie down. Separate the limbs. Then wrap the dry sheet and blankets around your body.

11. The "authentic" method is to first place the wet sheet from the sink on the bed before going into bath. Then wrap your body in large towels, put on slippers, discard the towels, and quickly lie down on the bed on the cold damp sheet with your arms upraised. As rapidly as possible, bring the right half of the wet sheet over the trunk and right leg. Tuck it in, and lay the loose folds between the legs. Lower the arms. Bring the left half of the sheet over the front of your body. Cover your shoulders, trunk, arms, and left leg. Turn on your left side, and the sheet goes under the right side. Turn up any excess.

Pin the cotton sheet so that no air can emerge. It should be snug, but not tight. Do not let two skin surfaces touch. The sheet is between the skin and the blanket. Next, fold the blankets snugly over your body in envelope fashion.

If you feel feeble, place a hot water bottle on your feet to speed the reaction. Additional light covers may also be added to speed the reaction. They can be applied from chin to ankles, *but do not cover the feet.* Tuck in around shoulders, and remove extra blankets as soon as the heat reaction occurs.

For *very nervous* persons who cannot bear the thought of being wrapped up, use a less extensive pack up to the armpits. The arms are left free. This three-quarter or half pack will have many of the same results as the full pack. If the patient has no heat reaction or gets cold, take pack off, cover the patient, and place hot water bottles at feet.

During a high fever, leave the pack on for 10 to 30 minutes, and reapply it later. If you are using the pack to relieve excessive menopausal heat, leave it on for 20 minutes to several hours. The pack may be left on overnight, particularly when you are attempting to avert a potential illness.

DAMP COLD SHEET PACK
(or Cold Double Body Compress)

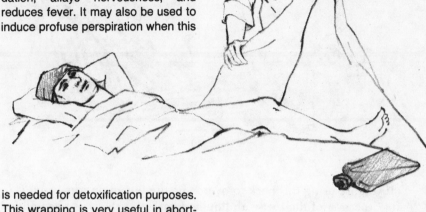

Fig. 18. This cold sheet wrapping, with body encased mummy-fashion in a series of dry sheets and blankets, is one of the most powerful of water therapy techniques. It is useful for sedation, allays nervousness, and reduces fever. It may also be used to induce profuse perspiration when this

is needed for detoxification purposes. This wrapping is very useful in aborting a cold or flu, and can be an effective aid in many chronic diseases, as it draws stored poisons out of the body.

Note the wrapping is similar to the simple cold double throat compress. Make sure that the feet don't touch, and that the arms are wrapped separately away from the body. The outer dry sheet and wool blanket prevent air from cooling the body, and the body heats the wet sheet from within. This acts as a heating compress, and that is why the patient feels so comfortable in a short time. However, since the encased arms can make some pa-

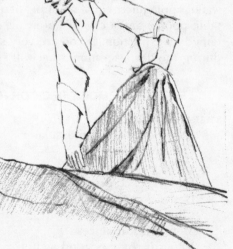

tients uneasy for a while, stay with them until they fall asleep. The compress can also be used in a shorter ¾ or ½ body compress in which the arms are left out, but covered with a light blanket.

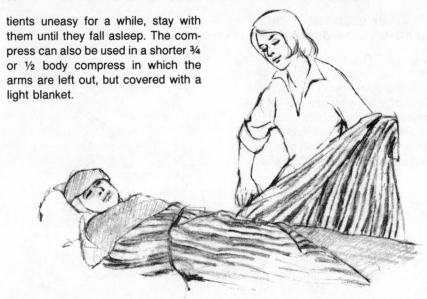

If you are using this pack to overcome the flu, an optional step is to "paint" the *soles* of the feet with liquified garlic tea that has been added to some heavy cold cream or vaseline. Then put white cotton socks over the feet, and put the feet *under the wet sheet,* and covered by the dry sheet and the blankets.

End the application by sponging your body with diluted apple cider vinegar. Do this in sections so that you do not become chilled. Dry, using a coarse towel. Change the bed linens.

Since this is a perspiration-inducing technique, and is not energizing, you should then go back to bed. Sip diluted apple cider vinegar and water; apple juice; equal amounts of apple cider vinegar and honey (1–3 tablespoons) and a cup of water; or, if desired, any vegetable juice obtained by extraction. If you are very sick, stick to only one type of juice during the day, as a mono diet will speed the healing.

HOT MOIST PACK OR HOT BLANKET PACK

THERAPEUTIC USES

Chronic joint and muscular
    rheumatism
Children's diseases
Children's convulsions
Gout
Chronic neuralgia
Mental disturbances
Nephritis (not as good as hot
    half baths)

Sciatica
Kidney stones
Blood poisoning
To create profuse
    perspiration
To elevate body
    temperature

This pack is applied in the same way as the damp sheet pack except that the cotton or linen sheet or blanket (preferred) is plunged into 110°F *hot* water. Wring dry, as a very wet blanket loses heat too quickly.

Similar hot packs can be devised for any area of the body. These partial packs help to shunt blood into other areas to break up congestion.

The value of the hot moist pack is that it induces perspiration very quickly, and thus helps eliminate toxic material through the skin. It also decreases internal congestion. Cotton and linen packs are used for children and feeble persons, but the blankets retain the heat longer than the cotton, and can be used whenever sustained heat action is needed.

The warm moist pack was used by Dr. J. H. Kellogg to hasten the release of toxins in children's diseases. He considered it more valuable in combating children's diseases than any drug.

Method

1. Prepare an ice bag, several hot water bottles, and a blanket or sheet to steep in the hot water.

2. Prepare the bed with protective material. It is useful, but not entirely necessary, to first use a rubber or plastic sheet. Over this, place 2 small blankets, or one very large blanket. The blanket should be large enough to overlap the edge of the bed, reach to your neck, and still have room at the bottom to turn up like an envelope.

3. Use either a large cotton (or linen) sheet, or an old soft wool blanket. Fold the blanket (or sheet) in thirds, then lengthwise. Holding the ends, immerse it into an extremely hot water bath. Use rubber gloves to wring or squeeze out all of the water.

4. Place the wrung-out blanket or sheet over the dry blankets on the bed, and lie on the bed on your back with *arms upraised.*

5. Apply a cold compress to the forehead and place an ice bag wrapped in a dish towel on your heart.

6. Wrap the wet blanket over the right side of your body. Bring your arms down and quickly drape the left side of the wet blanket over the front of the body.

7. Wrap the dry blanket(s) over the wet one, tucking it in at the shoulders and the feet. If there is a large rubber or plastic sheet underneath the dry blankets, bring it up and tuck it in at this time (it will help retain the heat longer, and cause additional perspiration).

8. Place a series of hot water bottles at the feet, and along the sides of the body.

9. Drink copious amounts of water or herb drinks.

10. Continuously replace the forehead compress so that it is always cold.

This pack can be applied from 5 to 20 minutes, depending on your health. The results are so pleasant that you will want to repeat it often, but too many treatments will make you feel exhausted.

There is a danger of becoming chilled when the covers are removed, so remove them in the following manner: Slide out the hot water bottles, the ice bag, the wet blankets and rubber sheet, and have a helper slide in a large, dry, warm sheet. Make sure you are continuously covered with the dry blanket. Rub the warm sheet gently over your entire body to get dry. Replace this sheet (it will be damp) with a dry one. Apply another hot water bottle to the feet. Rest or sleep for several hours.

This pack relaxes and soothes the muscles and helps to eliminate toxins and eruptions. *It does, however, increase the body temperature and the pulse rate. The pulse rate must be watched—especially with children and feeble persons. If it increases too rapidly, end the procedure. Heart patients, diabetics, persons with arteriosclerosis or TB, or excessively feeble or aged persons should not use this pack.*

DRY BLANKET PACK

THERAPEUTIC USES

To induce perspiration	In coma
In shock	For chronic rheumatism
In collapse after hemorrhage	

The dry blanket pack is Preissnitz's original preparation for creating perspiration and inducing the elimination of liquids. It is an indispensible aid in reviving someone from a coma, and a valuable therapy for chronic rheumatism (the dry pack, unlike the hot moist pack, does *not* make you feel weak). This very simple wrapping produces a powerful reaction.

Method

Prepare the bed with two blankets—one on top of the other. If desired, a dry sheet can be placed on top.

Prepare a hot water bottle. This is especially useful for feeble patients, or those who will need a boost in heating the body.

Prepare hot lemonade, or any of these hot herbal teas: peppermint, thyme, sage, red raspberry. Small amounts of yarrow may be added. Use ⅛ to ¼ teaspoon of cayenne pepper tea added to a cup of boiling water to help control internal hemorrhaging.

Void bladder.

Take a 15 to 30 minute hot bath or hot footbath. Apply a cold compress to the forehead.

Tuck the blanket (or if a sheet is also used, tuck the sheet, and then the blanket) around the body. To increase perspiration, apply hot water bottles to the soles of the feet and the sides of the body.

Rest in a warm, well-ventilated room for a half hour. If there is a free flow of perspiration, apply a cold compress to the head.

Sponge the body with cold water, or immerse the entire body in a full cold bath for 30 seconds to 1 minute. Vigorously dry the body with a large coarse towel, and go back to bed. A refreshing sleep follows quickly, symptoms lessen, and you will generally show a marked improvement.

Do not use the pack if eruptive diseases (measles, scarlet fever, chicken pox, and the like), diabetes, arteriosclerosis, or cardiac weakness are present, or if you are excessively nervous.

MUSTARD PACK
(or Mustard Plaster)

THERAPEUTIC USES

Break up internal congestion	Lumbago
Relieve pain	Neuritis
Improve local circulation	Bronchitis
Act as counterirritant	Sciatica
Alleviate gout	

This is one of my favorite plant packs. Mustard powder (plus a touch of water and flour), when made into a paste and applied in a cloth on a lightly oiled skin, has the unique power of bringing blood to the surface of the skin. It quickly heats up the area, and, as the blood rushes to the skin surface, even the worst congestion diminishes.

Method

Prepare some paper toweling, and a large linen or cotton dish towel. Fold the cloth in thirds. In a separate bowl, mix 1 tablespoon of dry, powdered (not hot) mustard with 4 to 8 tablespoons of flour. The less flour, the stronger the effect. To make the pack stronger, use equal amounts of mustard and flour. Double and triple the amounts according to the size poultice needed. Moisten the mixture with tepid water (hot water prevents the release of the needed oils) until it has the consistency of cream cheese.

Place the mustard paste on the paper toweling. Fold the toweling to make a packet, and place it in the folded dish cloth, or clean folded cotton cloth. Heat the pack by placing it on a hot water bottle.

If you have sensitive skin, oil the skin lightly with olive or vegetable oil. Place a thin cloth such as a large man's handkerchief on the area, and apply the mustard pack (or plaster). Cover the area with a blanket.

At first the heat may seem intense, but then it lessens, and, in my experience, always seems merely hot. As the skin becomes very red, the pack can be transferred from area to area, from the front of the chest to the upper back (for bronchitis) or on areas of intense pain.

Apply the pack to each area for 2 to 10 minutes. The entire treatment should last a half hour. After this, the pack loses its potency.

EARTH PACKS

THERAPEUTIC USES

Rheumatic problems	Neuralgia
Pain	Arthritis
Burns	Chronic joint inflammation
Stings	Muscle spasms

Chronic sciatica   To neutralize toxins
Gout

Hot sand, hot mud packs, and clay packs have been used for centuries by different cultures to relieve joint pain. The material used is either organic volcanic ash, peat from bogs, mineral sea mud, or clay from high mineral areas. All of these substances are available in powder form. For ordinary household first aid, I keep an inexpensive 5-pound ball of *neutral* Jordan clay ready in a closed container.

Clay packs have extracting ability because the mineral content increases the heat and chemical action on the skin. Because clay and/or earth draw out poisons, such packs not only soften the skin and release tension around joints, but also absorb internal toxic or pathogenic material.

The Cattier Company of France makes several excellent, neutral green-clay products including powdered green clay, clay toothpaste, clay soap, and clay masks. Weleda sells an excellent internal and external clay (Luvos #1, #2). Pottery firms, or firms that service rehabilitation departments in hospitals or spas, may be a source of other therapeutic earth substances.

Method

Heat up the clay or mud in a large double boiler. Add pure mineral or spring water to soften it. Spread this in one or two-inch thicknesses on a soft cotton cloth, slightly larger than the area you wish to cover. Place the hot clay or mud directly on the hurt area. Cover the area with a dry lightweight cloth. Leave on until it dries (15–30 minutes). Rinse off with warm water, then splash with a little cool water.

When an area is inflamed, or hot, as in a burn, use cold "chunks" of moistened clay to extract the heat. Envelop the area in a *thick* layer of wet clay, and the pain will seem to disappear. Next, cover the area with plastic or oilskin to keep it moist.

In the case of a severe burn, however, it is imperative to see a physician.

Earth packs can also be made by adding layer upon layer of the hot (or cold) clay *directly* on the skin. Or the hot "mud" can be placed in a small cotton pillow case with an "open window" and applied *directly* to the area. I used just such an application of cold mud to neutralize and detoxify my body during a case of food poisoning.

Remove the dried mud by sponging the flakes off, and then taking a needle shower. Dry gently with a mild cloth. If the body is still heated, keep the area warm and dry afterward.

Small applications of clay or mud will vitalize almost any area, *but do not take large baths in mud if you have heart disease, diabetes, high blood pressure, or arteriosclerosis.*

(13)

Showers

A shower is a directed stream of water used on one area or the whole body. The temperature, shape, and force of each shower determines its healing and physiological effect.

Showers can be *rain* or *fan* (gentle, dispersed stream with low pressure) or *jet* or *percussion* (powerful, direct stream with great pressure) and are used in cold, hot, neutral, or alternating temperatures. A dousing shower is one poured from a pail or a great height.

COLD SHOWER

THERAPEUTIC USES

As a tonic

To reduce high temperatures

To overcome fatigue

To overcome collapse

Use water that is as cold as you can tolerate. Remain in the shower for at least several seconds. Your endurance to the cold will increase as you do this regularly.

HOT SHOWER

THERAPEUTIC USES

Prepare a patient for
  a cold treatment

Alleviate pain

Sedate central nervous system

Soothe irritated skin

A light rain shower eases neuralgic pains, and will alleviate the discomfort of hives and itching. During a very hot shower, prevent a headache or dizziness by applying a cold compress on the forehead and neck.

Duration: 30 seconds to 2 minutes. 100°F–104°F.

NEUTRAL SHOWER

THERAPEUTIC USES

    Pelvic problems   Nervousness   Bedwetting

A light, gentle fan or spray shower in *lukewarm*, body-temperature water will relax and calm the body by contracting the brain blood vessels. It acts in the same way as a long neutral bath. Neutral showers are useful for seminal weakness, bedwetting, and some cases of painful vaginal spasm.

Water temperature: 92°F–97°F.

Duration: 4–6 minutes.

ALTERNATE HOT AND COLD SHOWER

Because of their varied uses, alternate hot and cold applications may be the most important of the healing showers. There are two types of alternate hot and cold showers:

1. *Equal* amounts of hot and cold water.
2. *Unequal* amounts, with emphasis on the hot stream.

Equal: Alternate Hot and Cold

THERAPEUTIC USES

    Muscular rheumatism

    Stiff joints (if no inflammation of nerve)

    Enlargement of liver

Direct water on body or local area, 15 seconds hot, then 15 seconds cold.

Unequal: Longer Hot, Shorter Cold (Scots Shower)

THERAPEUTIC USES

Whole body: Muscle fatigue

             Lack of energy

             Profuse or frequent sweating

Local: Poor circulation

      Chronic backache

      Spinal irritations

      Uterine and ovarian neuralgia

      Gastric ulcer

      Congestion of the brain (when used on feet alone)

This is my favorite of all showers, for it has a remarkable and tonic effect on the body. This Scots shower is excellent for the circulation, and when used over a long period of time tends to affirm circulatory changes. It achieves the circulatory effect of an extreme, short cold-water treatment without producing any internal heat reaction within the body.

Use hot jet spray for 1–4 minutes. Follow immediately with a cold jet spray for 5 to 30 seconds.

If the cold spray is used for less than 10 seconds (but no less than 5 seconds), the general effect is one of increased circulation and sedation.

If the cold spray is used for more than 10 seconds (but no longer than 30 seconds), the body feels tonified and stimulated.

Special Uses of Unequal Alternate Hot and Cold Showers

THERAPEUTIC USES

Dry skin	Gastrointestinal catarrh
Profuse sweating	Congestion of liver and spleen
Cardiac inefficiency	Inflammation of uterus
Chronic gastritis	

Use streams of warm to hot water on areas that need stimulation. Gradually increase the heat, depending on your tolerance.

Use heat for 1–2 minutes or until the skin is cherry color. Follow with cold spray for 2–3 seconds.

LOCAL SHOWERS
(to one area)

Showers directed to only one part of the body can affect other parts of the body by reflex, or by diverting blood from that area.

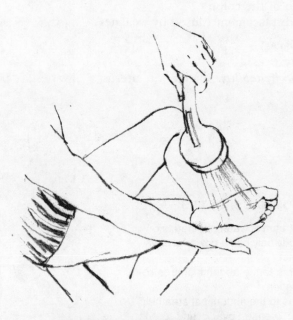

SOLES OF THE FEET SHOWER

Fig. 19. A stream of water directed to the soles of the feet can create a powerful physical effect. Such streams not only increase circulation, but also act either by diverting blood from another part of the body, and therefore relieving congestion somewhere else, or as a reflex connection to another organ, since there are so many reflex points on the soles of the feet. For more information on such water therapy, see Foot Baths and Feet.

SOLES OF FEET

THERAPEUTIC USES

Cold feet   Ejaculation of sperm because
Weakness of bladder   of relaxed condition
Incontinence of old persons

Use strong cold jet stream for ½ minute to 2 minutes.

ENTIRE FOOT

THERAPEUTIC USES

Prevents headaches

A cold broken jet or spray shower on the feet at the end of any shower contracts the blood vessels of the brain, and relieves any congestion in the head.

ABDOMEN

Cold (a few seconds)
THERAPEUTIC USES

Constipation
Dilation of the colon
Pelvic displacement caused by weakness

Hot (3–5 minutes)
THERAPEUTIC USES
For pain and irritability: bladder   uterus   ovaries   pelvic area

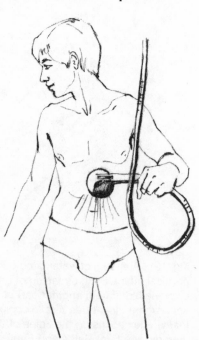

ABDOMINAL SHOWERS

Fig. 20.   A stream of water directed to one part of the body only has a powerful physiological impact.

Cold streams to the abdominal area relieve constipation.

Hot streams to the abdominal area help with bladder, uterine, ovary, and pelvic area pain and discomfort.

Alternate hot and cold streams to this area relieve chronic diarrhea and digestive problems, and may help with lower back problems.

Also see Abdominal Compress (pp. 38-39).

Alternate Hot and Cold (3 minutes hot; 30 seconds cold. Repeat several times.)

THERAPEUTIC USES
  Relieve irritation in lower back
  Tone abdominal organs
  Help to overcome chronic diarrhea

CHEST
(fan spray shower)

Cold (a few seconds)

THERAPEUTIC USES
To top, side, or back of chest: Increase flow of blood to skin,
                                muscles, and lungs
To breast: Stimulate blood to pelvis
          Contract muscles of the uterus

Prolonged Cold (2 minutes)

THERAPEUTIC USES
To chest: Contract the blood vessels of the lungs,
          lessen blood to that organ.
To breast: Contract the blood vessels of the uterus
          and relieve uterine congestion
To breastbone (lower sternum): Contract kidney vessels, increase
                                the flow of urine

SHOULDER
(jet shower)

THERAPEUTIC USES
  Constipation   Delay in development of young women
  Bladder troubles   Absence or abnormal stopping of
  Incontinence   menstrual period

A short cold shoulder shower (one minute) followed by a three-minute very hot shower (113°F and up) acts on the pelvic area and all other lower extremities through reflex action.

FACE AND SCALP
An application of very cold water on any part of the skin produces an excitant effect on the brain. A prolonged cold shower relieves congestion, while a short cold shower increases activity in the area. A neutral face and scalp shower relieves tension and excitement.

UPWARD PELVIC FLOOR AND ANUS
To obtain Bidet attachments for upward showers, see Resource List.

Cold

THERAPEUTIC USES

To anus only: Useful for hemorrhoids and constipation
For women: Upward shower acts on bladder, fallopian tubes
For men: Upward shower acts on prostate, ejaculatory ducts,
         testicles, bladder, pelvis, deep urethra

Hot

THERAPEUTIC USES

Rectal ulcers, fissures

This hot upward shower should end with several seconds of cold spray.

DOUSING SHOWER

THERAPEUTIC USES

High fevers   Hysteria
Sunstroke   Agitation of mentally
Children's diseases (when   disturbed
   air passages are clogged)   Asphyxiation
Scarlatina

The pouring of *cold* water over the body sharply awakens the vital forces. Such a shower is excellent for eliminating unnatural body heat (from fever and sunstroke), and for stimulating breathing. If you are treating someone who is in an alcoholic stupor, make sure to *rub their body* afterward with a towel to avoid secondary complications. If the skin of the person you are treating is exceptionally cold (as with nearly drowned persons), apply a hot water bottle or hot water to get the body more active.

A *neutral* temperature dousing that is directed to the spine, arm, foot, or feet has a *sedative* effect.

Do not use dousing if heart or kidney problems are present, or if there is any internal bleeding.

Method

Have a large sheet ready for rubbing the body. This is very important both to sharpen the effect of the application and to avoid secondary complications.

Wrap a cold towel around the patient's head. Pour water from as great a height as possible. The patient can stand or sit in tub with his hands crossed over the chest. The treatment can also be combined with the patient sitting in a hot water bath. Direct the first pailful of water to the *chest,* the second to the *back.* Rub trunk and limbs with a large dry sheet for 20 seconds. Wrap the patient in the sheet, and rub until the entire body is dry.

ENEMA

THERAPEUTIC USES

Eject waste materials from the lower bowel
Evacuate fecal material from the lower colon
Create kidney activity in disease states
Lower the temperature in fever
Stimulate the liver
Relieve irritation, pain in rectum
Relieve inflammation in rectum
Control diarrhea
Help with painful periods
Reduce pain in acute pelvic conditions
Reduce abdominal inflammation
Relieve cystitis

An enema is an injection of water into the rectum.

Method

To use such an irrigation, obtain a rubber gravity (fountain) syringe at the drugstore. Close the valve controlling the tube, and fill with several cups of water. Warm water is used in most evacuations, cold water is used in fever, and hot water is used to stimulate the body during certain health problems or diseases. Use 2 pints of water for adults; ½ to 1 pint for children, according to age. Five tablespoons of pure, undiluted coffee added to a quart of water is detoxifying and may be used when necessary. Chamomile tea will help reduce internal spasms. Catnip tea will relieve spasms and constipation.

Attach the rubber bottle to a hook about 4½ to 5 feet high on the wall or on the bathroom door. Lubricate the nozzle with cream, but make sure to keep nozzle holes open. Although an enema may be taken while sitting upright on the toilet, the best position is the knee-chest position on the floor. This changes the entire position of the bowel and colon, and water can penetrate into the body for quite a distance. If it is more convenient, take the enema while lying on the floor on your left side.

Insert nozzle into the rectum, open pressure clip, eliminate the air, and allow the water to flow into the body. Try not to let in air as this can be uncomfortable. Stop the water flow by pinching the rubber tube. Rub your abdomen in a clockwise fashion. This allows you to retain the water comfortably for a longer period of time.

Hot rectal irrigation is useful in painful cystitis, rectal spasm, and rectal pain, hemorrhoidal pain, in expelling gas, controlling gas, and relieving pelvic pain and will stimulate kidney function even where all drugs fail. *Cold* enemas stimulate the bowel profoundly, and can be used to shrink hemorrhoids, help reduce fever, and help the body throw off a cold. (See the listings in Part III.)

In treating chronic colitis, use a honey or molasses enema for its purging effect in reducing mucus and loosening hardened accumulations of mucus.

Enemas must not be used too often, as the body can lose its tone and ability to evacuate normally. When traveling, or for postoperative constipation, "Fleet" enemas can be used. They are available in sizes for adults and children, and can be purchased at drugstores.

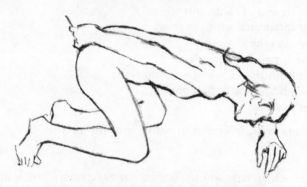

KNEE-CHEST POSITION FOR ENEMA

Fig. 21. An upward shower irrigation with a fountain syringe is effective in cleansing the lower bowel. This assists in the evacuation of stored waste material. An enema in the above knee-chest position allows the water stream to reach a larger portion of the colon than a sitting or lying position.

Internal irrigations should be used when fasting, to speed release of damaged and dying cells. Enemas evacuate poisons, bacteria, and virus in diarrhea, alleviate menstrual constipation and digestive problems, stimulate sluggish organs, are an integral part of detoxification programs, and can help to overcome some chronic disease problems. Herbal teas and lactic acid substances may be added to the enema when needed to restore internal flora or control spasms.

VAGINAL DOUCHE

A vaginal douche is an irrigation of the vaginal area with water, or medicated remedy, such as rosemary tea.

THERAPEUTIC USES

Relieve itching

Overcome yeast infection

Overcome white discharge

Relieve pain

Relieve spasm

Help control pain or flow before period

Purchase a special hand vaginal spray, or use the long spray nozzle available with all fountain syringes. This can be attached to the wall. The water flows in by gravity.

Method

Fill the bag with plain water, or medicated water as described under "Vagina," pages 216–217. Sit on toilet or sit in bathtub and let the water flow in and out of the bulb syringe or nozzle.

Weak rosemary tea douches can be used for a week or so to overcome many vaginal and ovarian problems. Use a tablespoon to a cup of boiling water. Steep the rosemary for 20 minutes, strain, and add to a quart-sized douche bag.

Normally, the vaginal cavity should *not* be douched too often, because irrigation eliminates normal body acidity.

HOW TO CLASSIFY WATER TEMPERATURE

	Fahrenheit	Centigrade
VERY COLD	32°F–56°	0°C–13.3°
COLD	56°F–65°	13.3°C–18.3°
COOL	65°F–75°	18.3°C–23.9°
TEPID	75°F–92°	23.9°C–33.3°
NEUTRAL	92°F–98°	33.3°C–36.1°
WARM TO HOT	98°F–104°	36.1°C–40°
VERY HOT	104° and above	40° and above

WHEN YOU DON'T HAVE A THERMOMETER

To achieve a hot bath you will need 1 quart of hot boiling water for every 2 quarts of cold water. Place the cold water in the bath first and add the hot water in order not to lose the heat. Use the same proportion for gallons of water.

WHEN YOU DON'T HAVE THERMOMETER

COLD WATER 53°F	BOILING WATER 212°F	BATHWATER
2 quarts	1 quart	3 quarts 106°F
2½ quarts	1 quart	3½ quarts 98°F
3 quarts	1 quart	4 quarts 93°F
4 quarts	1 quart	5 quarts 85°F
5 quarts	1 quart	6 quarts 80°F
6 quarts	1 quart	7 quarts 76°F
8 quarts	1 quart	9 quarts 71°F

To gradually increase the water temperature of a bath by 1°F at a time, remove one cupful of the bathwater, and add two cups of very hot or boiling water.

Each replacement *increases* the bath temperature by 1°F.

(14)

Techniques
for Children

Most of the techniques in this book are suitable for children, and some
of the quickest and most enthusiastic responses to the washes, wrappings,
and cold friction massage may come from the children in your life. Naturally, as in all activities with children, you must be able to judge reaction
and timing. If a child resists some of the cold water therapies, don't force
them, but gradually introduce them some other time.

*It is a good idea to consult your child's pediatrician about the suitability of any
one procedure.*

If you feel a child is getting sick, it is most important to quickly
detoxify the body. This is accomplished by sweating and flushing the
system. Follow the directions for any of the perspiration procedures, or
take this shortcut: Give the child herbal tea, place him or her in a nightgown or pajamas, and zip the child into a sleeping bag for a long and
comfortable sleep. The child will awaken soggy with perspiration, but
almost free of the bacterial or viral infection (providing you have caught
it in its early stage). Wash the child, and change his or her clothes. More
often than not, a healthy child will have overcome the indisposition, and
will be able to go back to play almost immediately.

Anti-sore throat compresses, and the many partial or full baths used
to abort colds or other minor indispositions, are of special interest for
children. There are innumerable effective first-aid hints throughout this
book, including the use of ice or compresses for specific injuries, or apple
cider vinegar washes for various sprains and strains. Neutral baths will
help to sedate an overactive or tense child, while the many cold water
treadings and splashes will help your child develop a tolerance to cold
water, and a resistance to disease. Thyme tea baths will also help to

strengthen a weak child. Chamomile, linden, or fennel tea will help with most children's digestive problems.

The salt solution washes and body dips mentioned in this book help to shorten any eruptive disease, and are useful in measles, chicken pox, scarlatina, and scarlet fever.

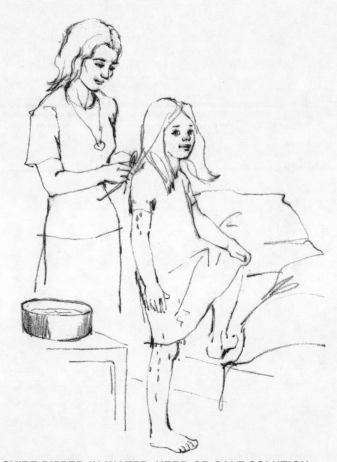

SHIRT DIPPED IN WATER, HERB OR SALT SOLUTION

Fig. 22. This shortcut body compress has the same effect as any cold double compress, and will generate internal heat. This induces perspiration, and helps the child to throw off stored toxins, reduce fever, or bring eruptive diseases to a quick end.

Prepare the bed with some protective covering. Place a large blanket over the bed and several dry sheets over the blanket. Dip the shirt into either a salt solution, apple cider vinegar, cold water, or herb solution according to the health need. Place immediately over the child and rush the child into bed. First wrap the top dry sheets around the child, and then encase the child in the blanket. If the child is uncomfortable in such a wrapping, place a dry sheet over the body, and cover that sheet with a larger, light down comforter or wool blanket. Once the comforter is in place the child will start to warm up and feel very drowsy and comfortable.

Kneipp's special technique: Dissolve a cup or two of table salt in two quarts of cold water. Wash the child with this water, or put a long cotton shirt on the child, and dip the child in the water. Then put the child to bed, or apply salt-dipped compresses to the eruptive area. This technique will not only shorten the duration of any eruptive disease, but lessen the impact.

PART III

Water Works:
Health Problems
and
Water Therapy

Once the techniques of water therapy have been mastered, they can then be applied to a wide variety of ailments. The following are the *specific* therapeutic uses of water. As stated earlier, test and check each step in any of these procedures to ensure personal safety.

ACNE

Water Therapy

Pure water is essential in cleansing the system. Drink two or three glasses of pure, cold water on arising. Also drink vegetable juices, carrot juice, and such herbal teas as chamomile, red clover, peppermint, and nettle, or nettle juice.

Facials

It is important to keep the skin of the face as clean as possible. Do not touch the face with your hands, and control blackheads and whiteheads by frequently steaming the face. This opens the pores, and blackheads may be gently released with cotton swabs.

For directions, see page 60.

Acne Scars

Combine powdered marigold (pot marigold-calendula) petals and honey, or 1 teaspoon of powdered nutmeg and honey, or nutmeg and vitamin E oil. Daub on the scars with your fingertips. Allow to dry for 20 minutes. Then rinse with warm water and splash face with cool water. Use once a week to reduce acne scars.

General Therapy

Eliminate junk foods, exercise regularly, and breathe lots of fresh air. Walk in the sunshine for a few minutes each day. Meditate to overcome stress.

Using antibiotics lessens your future immunity, and destroys natural intestinal flora. Moreover, they don't get to the cause of the acne problem, but merely hide it temporarily. Years from now, you will regret utilizing an antibiotic for this purpose.

ACHILLES TENDON

Water Therapy

Whirlpool therapy and plunging the feet in alternate hot and cold foot baths will increase the circulation. Treading in cold water will also strengthen the feet, and help tone up the entire body. Water treatment is an adjunct to general therapy.

General Therapy

Athletes know that taping around the heel that is too tight sometimes produces a strain in the Achilles tendon. Other times, the strain is caused by one side of the body being higher than another. This imbalance is easily adjusted by a professional chiropractor or osteopath. Also, a heel lift will help to balance the unequal sides of the body.

ADENOIDS

Water Therapy

Walk and wade in cold water up to your calves.

Irrigate your nose by washing each nostril internally with either a salt solution or a mild horsetail (herb) tea. There is a professional nose irrigator spray which can be attached to a Water Pik. See Resource List.

Use an ice "collar" frequently. Dip a rolled towel into ice water, wring out, and wrap around the neck. Professional ice bag collars are available from rehabilitation sources, or neck-shaped hydrocollator cold packs may be used.

ANKLE

WEAK ANKLES

Water Therapy

Tread in cold water as often as possible.

Frequently plunge the feet into alternate hot and cold foot baths.

SPRAIN

Water Therapy

Minor sprain: An initial hour of ice therapy and elevation reduces swelling and tenderness. Afterward, use Gibney taping, and every several hours strap the ice bag over the taping with an elastic bandage. The ankle will need continuous elevation. Do a minimum of walking. Use a raw onion wrap over the ankle during the night to reduce pain and swelling. Apple cider vinegar wrappings are also helpful.

Major Sprain: Follow the same instructions of taping, compression, ice therapy, and elevation. Prevent further swelling and internal bleeding by bed rest. As above, raw onion or apple cider vinegar wrappings are helpful.

Rehabilitation

The following hot and cold foot bath, suggested by Sayers "Bud" Miller, Athletic Coordinator, Pennsylvania State University, is excellent rehabilitation therapy for sprains.

Note: This is one of the rare applications that *ends with hot water.* Most alternate applications must end with cold water, and most hot water treatments are followed by a toning with cold water.

FOREFOOT (below the ankle sprain)

The area *below the ankle* is the calcaneocuboid, an area often twisted or turned in daily life and in sports.

Water Therapy

Use ice therapy immediately. Attach the ice bag with an elastic bandage to produce compression, and elevate the foot. The time required for rehabilitation depends on the age and fragility of the patient. Most athletes will be able to walk without pain within 2–3 days.

General Therapy

Use a figure 8 strapping, and continue for 2 weeks.

I like arnica lotion for such pain, and apply it directly to the pained area.

BONE BRUISE ON ANKLE

This area tends to be susceptible to bruises, and will remain tender after the first bruise.

Water Therapy

Attach an ice bag, placing another fabric between the ankle and the bag. Create some compression with an elastic bandage. Elevate the ankle area.

General Therapy

Generally, keeping off your feet for 24–48 hours helps to heal the bruise.

In sports, it is a good practice to attach a thin rubber padding on the outside of the shoe or skate to prevent further problems. If the strainlike pain persists, some trainers tape the ankle on a routine basis.

ANOREXIA
(loss of appetite)
Water Therapy

Apply an ice bag to the stomach for a half hour before meals to stimulate the digestive system.

Some loss of appetite occurs at the beginning of fevers and illnesses. In this case, the body *doesn't* require much food, and drinking liquids, especially water, is preferred.

The ice bag is helpful when loss of appetite is caused by nervousness, distaste for food, alcoholic excesses, and cocaine or other drug addiction.

APPENDICITIS

Water Therapy

Precede water treatment with an enema. *Never use a laxative.*

Simultaneous Treatment

Apply an ice bag over the appendix. This causes reflex contraction of the blood vessels. At the same time, *wrap the legs,* or the legs and hips, in a *hot* leg pack, or *hot* hip pack. This will relieve the pain instantly because it draws the blood from the inflamed part. Use these treatments for 30 minutes.

At the end of 30 minutes, rub all parts of the body *except the abdomen* with a cold mitten massage.

Thereafter, continuously apply ice bags to the inflammation.

If it is impossible to wrap the legs in hot packs, apply an ice bag over the appendix and cover it with a large hot moist compress.

Either treatment may be repeated as often as necessary to control the pain.

After the Acute Stage

After the temperature gets back to normal and the acute tenderness subsides (usually from 12–24 hours after the attack has started) apply alternate hot and cold compresses for 5 minutes at a time. Repeat several times for one day.

After this, avoid any further treatment to abdomen or appendix since it may cause peristalsis and enough internal activity to encourage additional inflammation, or rupture of the appendix.

ANEMIA
(iron deficiency)

Water Therapy

Initial treatment: Stimulate and warm the body with short hot compresses, followed by cold compresses, and apply to spine or abdomen. Alternate this treatment occasionally with a hot foot bath. After each treatment, vigorously tap and stroke the abdomen, and wash the area with cold water and friction massage. Do the same to the spinal area.

Later treatment: As the circulation in the body improves, also use alternate hot and cold gentle spray showers directed to the spine. As soon as possible graduate to a strong jet stream.

Also massage the body with the salt rub before taking occasional neutral baths (10 minutes).

General Therapy

Walk in fresh or, ideally, mountain air, and use Swedish massage therapy. Red cells are temporarily increased by massage, and the effect lasts longer as treatments are repeated.

See also "Digestive Problems," page 139.

ARCH SPASM

Water Therapy

Mild spasm: Attach an ice bag to the foot and arch area. Do not walk too much.

Severe spasm: Attach an ice bag with elastic bandages to provide compression, and walk with crutches.

General Therapy

Add an arch support to shoe to reduce further problems. See also "Feet," page 150.

ARM INJURIES

Ice therapy, with compression bandaging and elevation of the injured arm (if possible), is the usual initial treatment for arm injuries. Later, neutral arm baths will reduce congestion and quicken healing, and also lessen pain as well as formation of pus.

Arm area *spasms* should be treated with hot moist compresses.

BICEP STRAIN

In contact sports, the muscle under the biceps is greatly exposed and subject to repeated impact. This commonly leads to a contusion in the area.

Water Therapy

Apply ice bag and pressure bandaging to quiet the bruise.

Later soak the entire arm in apple cider vinegar and water, or apply diluted apple cider vinegar compresses.

General Therapy

Pad the bicep area after the first bruising, as the muscle under the bicep is very susceptible to additional bruising—especially with athletes —and repeated injury causes calcification.

"DEAD ARM"

The so-called "dead arm" is an acute and frightening experience that occurs in several sports, especially baseball. It is a result of a contusion to the arm that erupts suddenly in extreme radiating pain. "Dead arm" usually disappears in a few minutes, and rarely causes any permanent injury to the arm.

Water Therapy

Immediately apply several ice bags, or an ice pack made with a towel large enough to cover the entire arm.

General Therapy

Add padding to the arm. If the symptoms persist, see a physician.

ELBOW CUTS

A deeply penetrating laceration in the elbow often creates a secondary infection as well. This may result in a large swelling in the area.

Water Therapy

Wash the cut, and irrigate frequently in neutral-temperature elbow baths. Apply a local pressure bandage without drainage.

General Therapy

Immobilize the elbow in a sling for 8–10 days.

ELBOW STRAIN

Abnormal strain of the elbow (hyperextension) results in extreme tenderness and swelling.

Water Therapy

Immediately after the injury, apply ice to reduce the swelling.

General Therapy

After the initial ice therapy, place the elbow in a sling. These two therapies will reduce the swelling in 2–3 days.

Use an elbow cinch strapping to limit elbow extension. Gentle massage is also helpful. Use arnica lotion, or Olbas oil to massage and reduce pain.

The elbow must be completely healed before the athlete returns to competition. Many trainers advise working out with a 20-pound bar to regain range of motion.

FOREARM CONTUSION

This is a most common injury in contact sports, where impact with football helmets or contact with the cleats on athletic shoes can cause painful multiple lacerations, bruises, or contusions.

Water Therapy

Immediately apply ice bag to reduce internal bleeding. If there is no fracture, wrap the ice bag in elastic pressure bandage, and elevate the forearm with a sling. Afterward, use frequent neutral-temperature arm baths to speed healing and reduce the pain.

To further increase the circulation to the area, use these alternate hot and cold applications: hot and cold showers, hot and cold arm baths, hot and cold compresses.

FOREARM SPASM

This type of spasm frequently occurs to oarsmen.

Water Therapy

Apply hot moist compresses on the area of pain. Also frequently plunge the entire arm into a neutral arm bath.

General Therapy

A week of self-paced stroking in a single shell will offset the pain and spasm.

ARTERIES
(hardening)

Water Therapy

Drink large quantities of distilled water. This water has an affinity for the deposits of lime salts in the walls of the arteries and promotes their elimination.

Preventive Measure

On arising, take a 10-minute warm bath. Relax as thoroughly as you can and breathe deeply. Finish the treatment with a quick cold shower or cold sponging for 1–2 minutes.

The warm bath produces a moderate relaxation of tissues and blood vessels. The short cold applications produce a contraction with secondary dilation. By using the hot and cold in an *alternate fashion,* the blood vessels are exercised and good body tone and nutrition are augmented.

ARTHRITIS

Arthritis is a disease of the whole system, and responds to several coordinated therapies.

Water Therapy

Distilled water: Drink distilled water every morning. Distilled water is said to be very effective in reversing and controlling arthritis because it has an affinity for mineral salts and vegetable acids. This binding and attraction works to absorb and eliminate mineral salts and other waste products through the kidneys.

Raw potato juice: You can also drink a glass of raw potato juice every morning. Blend a clean raw potato and peel with an equal amount of water. To prepare without blending, cut the potato into slices and soak in a glass of water overnight.

Colon irrigation: An enema in a knee chest position will wash out accumulated poisons, and helps through osmosis in liquifying the bile. It also activates the sweat glands, and stimulates the kidneys.

To increase circulation: One of the best circulation builders is the cold mitten massage. Because this is a sectional massage, the inflamed joints never need to be touched. The body reacts well to the massage.

Short duration cold baths, cold half baths, and cold showers are excellent aids and will also help increase the circulation. Over the weeks and months, the showers can be made increasingly colder, and the pressure gradually increased. These various cold water techniques will promote the elimination of toxins retained in the joints.

Showers: Start the program with a gentle circular shower at 100°F, gradually cool the water to 90°F, and add considerable pressure.

This shower should be followed by a series of invigorating Scots showers of long hot streams (begin first with a warm stream) and *very short* cold streams alternately *played on the joints.*

Scots showers were researched in Germany by Professor Max Shuller, and reported to the XXI Surgical Congress. They diminish pain, increase mobility of the joints, and are particularly effective with ankle and wrist problems.

Perspiration: Perspiration helps eliminate toxic wastes from the body. Neutral baths (95°F) may be taken by robust arthritic patients to help them perspire and relax. For additional detoxification help, add either hayflower or oatstraw tea to the bath no more than 3 times a week.

Robust patients will also benefit from the dry hot pack, a body blanket pack. This pack must be followed by a sponging with tepid water and a light massage friction drying, or a full tepid bath that ends with cool water.

Pain and inflammation: Wrap and pin cold wet compresses around the swollen or tender joints. Cover the compress with a light cloth or flannel. The double compress may be left on all night if desired.

Other ways to help ease the pain: hot flaxseed poultice, mustard plaster or pack, paraffin bath.

Simmer the flaxseed in a nonaluminum bowl and place it steaming hot in a kitchen towel that has been folded several times. Apply it to the joints. See mustard pack page 93 and paraffin bath page 57.

General Therapy: Prevention

Many nutritional experts suggest a nonmeat diet with emphasis on raw vegetables and high potassium foods, especially avocados and pecans. Alkaline vegetables, including white potatoes, and raw vegetable juices, sour apples, pineapple, and bananas are all very helpful. Do *not* drink alcohol or coffee.

ASTHMA

Water Therapy

Children: Add two tablespoons of apple cider vinegar to a cup of warm water. Sponge the child with this solution, starting with the back and the chest. Expose only one part of the body at a time. Completely envelop the child in a light flannel blanket and put him to bed under light covers. The blanket "compress" will help the body to produce warmth, and the cramp will lessen. Follow these procedures for a week following the attack.

Also frequently bathe the child in full warm baths, and end each bath with a 1-second cold water dip.

Adults: Drink hot water and lemon juice each morning.

Strengthen the body with tonic measures.

Inhale steam and use tepid, fan shower sprays directed to the area below the ribs, to the pit of the stomach (midline), to the midline of the back, and the sides of the chest.

During an attack: Many water treatments will ease the constricting spasm. A herbal vapor tent will relieve the problem, but an even more effective treatment is a series of water treatments that act to draw blood away from the troubled area into another region of the body.

Several applications will accomplish this rerouting of the blood:

1. Apply an ice compress to the back of the head. Also take a hot footbath. Add mustard powder for additional effect.

2. Immerse hands in hot water for several seconds.

3. Apply a hot moist compress, an apple cider vinegar compress, or a hot hayflower compress over the entire bronchial area. When the compress loses its heat, wash the body with brisk sectional spongings. Replace the cloths every 15 minutes, or whenever cool.

4. If you cannot lie down for the chest application, apply the hot vinegar compress on the stomach and walk around. As soon as the warmth is generated in the stomach, it warms the chest and diverts the blood downward. This makes the pain more bearable and eventually removes it.

5. A hot enema is another procedure which is especially advised for asthma sufferers who have intestinal and kidney complications. Use the enema every half hour until the spasms stop.

Long Range Preventive Water Therapy

Cold treading: To strengthen and harden the body, walk in cold water up to the ankles or calves.

Vapor head bath: A steam vapor head bath in a warm, no-draft room has an important "dissolving" effect. Pour a quart or so of boiling water over any of these: bruised fennel seeds, linden flowers, sage leaves, elder flowers, yarrow, or nettle. Place the pot on a table, and improvise a tent around your head and the pot with an umbrella or towel. Close your eyes and breathe with your mouth open. Do not let any air in. Perspiration will flow in about 5 minutes.

In an emergency, this technique may be used every other day for a week. At other times, use only twice a week.

Half bath in tepid water: Ten-minute half baths with tepid water (80°F–85°F) have a tonic effect on the system. Wash first with tepid water, then sponge the upper back with cold water 3 times. Between each cold sponging, massage the chest and arms with a dry washcloth.

Breathing exercise: This deep exhalation exercise is excellent: Blow a feather or a small piece of paper across a wide table by exhaling deeply. The breathing in between exhalations should be normal. Repeat 10 times a day.

General Therapy

Asthma attacks are terrifying to both the sufferer and his or her family, and anxiety about an attack can aggravate another one.

There are several causes of attack. One type is initiated by sensitivity to pollen, molds, animal danders, lint, or insecticide. Another is caused by an infection in the nose, sinus, or lower lungs, and such attacks can be set off by changes in temperature, humidity, exposure to chemical, paint, or wax fumes. Others are caused by exhaustion, changes in endocrine balance during puberty, menstruation, pregnancy, and menopause. Many attacks are triggered by emotional stress.

Asthma sufferers should avoid the allergens they are sensitive to, and try not to become fatigued.

BACK
(lower back problems)

Water Therapy

The following two-part treatment will usually relieve acute lower back problems in a week to 2 weeks and mollify chronic cases when used for an extended period.

Apply alternate hot moist compresses to the lower back region. Whenever possible, dilute the water with hot apple cider vinegar. Follow this with an alternate hot and cold percussion shower on the area of pain.

This two-part treatment may be alternated with long baths in neutral temperature water. Follow bath with a cold mitten friction massage.

General Therapy

Chiropractic treatment, connective tissue massages, and stretching exercises to strengthen the area are all helpful.

There are some excellent herbal liniments that will bring up the blood and stimulate the skin. Arnica lotion or ointment is useful on unbroken skin. Olbas oil or ointment combines several stimulating herbs.

BED SORES

Water Therapy

Periodic cold compresses stimulate the area of friction.

Several water mattresses have been devised. They are usually called "flotation" systems. The water chambers are separated with longitudinal baffles to prevent excess water motion. Such mattresses work on the flotation principle, distributing the body weight evenly and reducing pressure on body contact points.

Calendula and plantain ointments will heal the area of pressure.

BEDWETTING

Water Therapy

Children: Dip the child in a cold water bath for 2–3 seconds every day.

Children over 4 years of age should tread in cold water up to the calves for 5 minutes every day.

Adults: Tread for 3–5 minutes in cold water up to the calves. This will bring results within a week. End each treatment with a short cold arm bath. Continue treatment to maintain the body tone and assure vitality.

Before bedtime, take an occasional 10-minute hot shallow (sit) bath and immediately alternate it with a brief cold sit bath. Dry the body, and go to bed immediately.

Weakened persons may drink ½ cup of yarrow tea in the morning and evening.

General Therapy

Dig the knuckles into the area of the lower back whenever there is pain.

See also "Kidney Problems," page 173, and "Bladder," page 118.

BIRTH
(see Childbirth and Pregnancy)

BITES
(see Stings)

BLADDER

Water Therapy

Reflex areas for the bladder are located in the inner surface of the thighs, the soles of the feet, hands, and abdomen. Water applied to any of these areas will affect the bladder.

To Increase Tone

Take a cold shower directed on the soles of the feet. This should last several seconds. A cold jet shower directed on hands or abdomen will also help.

Pain

To ease pain in the bladder, apply a hot hayflower compress on the abdomen and replace it with another as soon as it cools. Use a series of 3–4 compresses. Follow with cool sponging and friction massage of the abdomen.

Weakness of Bladder

Offset general weakness in the bladder with frequent cold fan (very low pressure) showers directed to the center of the body, from the pubic bone to the navel. This helps to contract the entire pelvic area.

Also strengthen the bladder with a cold jet shower directed at the soles of the feet.

Infection of the Bladder

Use a sea sponge. Lightly sponge entire body with warm water or apple cider vinegar and water.

Apply a hot hayflower compress to abdomen.

Drink horsetail tea frequently.

Take a cold shallow bath that lasts several seconds. Simultaneously direct a cold spray to the hip area.

BLISTER

Water Therapy

Prevention: As soon as you are aware of any localized friction burning on the foot or hands, place that part in cold water until the burning sensation stops. This technique, used by many athletic trainers, *prevents* blister formation. Trainers also use alum powder foot baths to harden the feet.

If the blister does form, massage the area with ice. Within a day this therapy reduces the excess fluid from the swelling, and overcomes area tenderness.

General Therapy

Prevention: Wear white cotton socks under woolen socks. Apply calendula or a lanolin-based ointment, on *irritated* spots. Use a moleskin to protect "hot" spots on the feet.

A good shoe fit is an absolute necessity, especially for sports activities. It also helps to break in shoes first.

Blister Under a Callus

Some athletes develop a blister under a callus. Be on the alert for these potentionally painful blisters, and prevent their formation with frequent epsom salt soaks. Scrape the hardened skin with an emery board file. Do not use a knife.

BLOOD POISONING

Some people are exceptionally susceptible to quick infections from scratches, cuts, and bruises, and thus have to be on the alert to avoid blood poisoning (septicemia).

Water Therapy

Fill two pails, one with extremely hot water, another with ice water, including pieces of ice. Immerse swollen foot or arm in the hot water for 2 minutes, and quickly follow with a 15-second immersion in the ice water. Keep changing for 30 minutes. Repeat 4–5 times a day depending on the seriousness of the infection. A disinfectant such as potassium permanganate can be added to the pails.

When this procedure is followed at the onset of the infection, it is exceptionally effective, and only requires a few days to restore the blood to normal.

The object of this therapy is to increase the circulation and renew the blood flowing through the infected part. Never allow an infection to get to a stage where red lines extend upward. If this happens, the infection has spread and requires the immediate attention of a physician.

BLOOD PRESSURE

High blood pressure can be increased by smoking, obesity, intake of salt, animal fats, and alcoholic beverages, and is linked to emotional upsets as well as other factors. Many doctors feel that too often drugs are prescribed for *mild* cases and they question the risk involved by using long-range drug therapy for such cases.

The decision not to take medication, however, should be made in consultation with your doctor.

Water Therapy

All persons with high blood pressure should drink 2 glasses of distilled water on rising. Do not eat for a half hour after this.

Drinking on an empty stomach stimulates the kidneys long after the excess water has been eliminated. This is important as the kidneys are the safety valves of the bloodstream, lowering the pressure, and eliminating the volume in the blood vessels. The lower the internal pressure in the blood vessels, the less difficulty the heart has in propelling the blood through the vessels.

A knee-chest enema, or a professional high colonic, acts as a diuretic to increase the flow of the urine. This drains the blood by lessening the bulk, and decreases the labor of the heart.

You can use any number of friction methods to stimulate the body to eliminate unneeded toxins. Dry brush the body with a rough wash cloth before baths, and brush the feet with a stiff, natural brush. Use cold friction massage and salt massage once a week.

General Therapy

Drink garlic tea as often as your social life will allow. This remedy is very effective in lowering the blood pressure. Watermelon fasts several days in a row also help the kidneys to flush out fluids.

Juice fasts, rice diets, and high potassium foods are helpful in rehabilitation. Do not drink coffee or alcohol, and exercise regularly. Meditation or biofeedback techniques will also help to lower the pressure.

BOILS

Preventive Measures

Use warm soaks in epsom salts, herbal or mineral baths, and wash the armpit, neck, chest, and buttocks with friction materials.

Water Therapy

In the early stages when the boil is merely a pimple, it can be aborted by simultaneously applying ice on the boil and a hot moist compress *over the ice.*

To increase circulation in the boil area: Use alternate hot and cold jet showers on the area of potential boil. Any alternate hot and cold application will help.

Children's boils: Use an ice cube to abort the boil, and for a week following apply a hayflower-dipped damp shirt every other night before the child goes to bed. Cover the child with a cotton sheet and blanket to avoid chills.

Every other day sponge the child's body using the sectional cold friction massage technique, or dip the child into a cold bath for several seconds at a time.

During the second week use these techniques every three days or so.

General Therapy

Several herbs such as cabbage can be used directly on the boil: wash, dry, and chop *white* cabbage leaves and place on gauze. Apply to boil. Attach overnight, or replace when warm. Cabbage has an affinity for pus. Repeat daily until boil is cleared.

Drink nettle juice or tea, or red clover or burdock tea to purify the blood. You can help to bring a boil to a head by taping a banana skin to the area. Honey can also be applied to boils, and is quite germicidal.

Do not touch boils with hands, and do not squeeze. This spreads the infection. Boils frequently occur in contact sports, especially after the first to third week of practice when the fall weather is hot. Boils often occur on the knee in football since this area has a high rate of abrasion and contact with dirt.

Boils also occur when you are temporarily run down or in poor health. If you are prone to boils, make sure your barber or hairdresser sterilizes the shears, and there is not constant friction, as from a collar. Add vitamin B supplements, fresh vegetables, and fresh fruits to your diet, and avoid excess refined carbohydrate and sugar.

If there doesn't seem to be any cause for the boils, *check your teeth and tonsils.* One youngster I know was ill with boils for years until they took out her tonsils and discovered a large hidden pocket of pus.

BRAIN CONGESTION
(see Head)

BREASTS

Water Therapy

For caked and hard breasts, or small cysts, apply vitamin E oil, or 8:1 wheat germ oil directly on the breasts. Also, frequently apply large hot moist compresses on each breast. End every hot application with a cool sponging.

General Therapy

Drink some 8:1 wheat germ oil every day, or take a small amount of vitamin E in capsule form. This procedure, used with the above water and oil therapy, is effective in controlling cyst formation.

BREATH
(bad breath)

Water Therapy

Drink large quantities of water and of peppermint tea. Add a pinch of anise, cinnamon, or caraway powder to the drinks.

General Therapy

Fasting on apples only for several days will cleanse the system.

BRONCHITIS
(acute)

Water Therapy

The aim of this water therapy is to unblock chest congestion and promote free circulation of the blood. This can be accomplished in these ways:

Primary therapies:

1. The easiest method is the *cold double chest compress.* For quick action, dip a large towel into cold water, wring it out, and apply it slightly dripping, directly to the throat, chest, and abdomen. Cover the wet towel with a slightly larger dry towel. Then, cover the towels and yourself with bedcovers.

Change the wet towel every 2 hours, except if there is a fever. In this case, change the towel every hour, and apply the compress from throat to knee.

2. The double compress may be used, or alternated, with a *triangular throat-chest compress.* See page 34.

3. A *mustard plaster* application will also help to break up deep congestion. See page 93.

4. Small amounts of *powdered ginger* can be added to vaseline or Vicks Vaporub to relieve chest tightness.

5. A *mustard powder* or *plain hot foot bath* will draw congestion away from the chest by diverting the blood flow to the feet. Ginger powder may also be added to the foot bath.

Secondary therapies:

1. Use an enema (knee-chest position) twice a day. This stimulates the liver, and helps the osmotic action of the water application.

2. A steam vaporizer placed under a large umbrella "tent" is useful in breaking up congestion and easing breathing.

Be careful to avoid burning, excess perspiration, and drafts.

Bronchitis of the Aged

Apply a *hot moist compress* over the bronchial area every 15 minutes to ease expectoration.

Other Water Therapies

Strengthen the body by *walking in cold water* for several minutes every day. Increase skin action and ability to discard internal impurities with frequent *cold spongings* and *friction massages.* Occasionally take an *epsom salt bath* and *salt massage.* Take frequent *warm baths,* and follow the baths with a gentle *cold spray*—as often as twice a day. Each evening before bed, apply the cold double *triangular kerchief compress* (it has a heating action). In the morning sponge the throat and chest with *apple cider vinegar* or *cold water,* and briskly rub the area dry.

Drink lots of *hot lemonade,* and large quantities of *hot water* or hot herbal teas to check the chronic cough and relieve the pain.

BRUISES

ABRASION

An abrasion is a minor injury in which the superficial layers of the skin are removed. This can increase the vulnerability of the exposed skin layers to secondary infection.

Water Therapy

Wash area with mild soap and warm water. Apply local *warm compress.*

General Therapy

After washing, apply a healing lotion or ointment. Herb ointments such as calendula have outstanding healing powers. A slice of onion has remarkable healing powers and may be applied to the bruise. Sage tea compresses help with most bruises and expedite healing.

CONTUSION

A contusion is an injury with internal bleeding but no broken skin. The amount of the bleeding and swelling depend more on the location of the contusion than the extent of the injury. Soft tissues swell easily and must be attended to immediately.

Water Therapy

Apply ice immediately to stop the bleeding and control inflammation. Place a piece of fabric on the skin, and attach an ice-filled rubber bag with elastic bandage to create a small amount of compression. Usually ice therapy is applied for 30 minutes, twice a day.

With superficial bruises, normal activity may be resumed fairly soon. *Never use heat on a contusion for the first 24–48 hours, as heat restarts bleeding, and provokes inflammation.*

HEMATOMA

Hematoma is a tissue injury that swells and collects blood. The blood collection swells the tissues and creates a severe inflammation and local tenderness within the body.

Water Therapy

Place a molded rubber pad on the injury, apply an ice bag, and attach the bag with an elastic bandage to provide a slight compression. Also note specific instructions for each injury.

General Therapy

The ice therapy is continued as directed for each injury. It is urgent to keep the blood collection at a minimum, and reduce possible inflammation and swelling. Continue padding and compression for 7–10 days after the initial ice treatment.

A slice of onion may be applied under the ice. It will help to reduce the swelling as well as the pain.

SPRAIN

A sprain is a trauma to a joint which causes pain and disability depending on the degree of injury to the ligaments. In a severe sprain, ligaments may be torn completely. The ankle joint is often sprained, as is the wrist or knee joint. See specific instructions for ankle, wrist, and knee.

Water Therapy

Applying ice to the sprain, or soaking the sprain in very cold water, helps to alleviate pain and prevent further swelling. Cold water compresses, with or without apple cider vinegar or witch hazel or arnica lotion may also be used. During rehabilitation, apply alternate hot and cold compresses and use whirlpool baths to increase circulation.

General Therapy

You can alternate apple cider vinegar, witch hazel, or arnica compresses or onion poultices, or onion and salt poultices, with the ice therapy. Onion slices may be applied directly to the sprain, and attached with a bandage. The onion and salt application has excellent results. Combine equal amounts of grated onion with salt to make a paste, and apply directly to injured area. Wrap with a bandage, and overwrap with an elastic bandage. Keep area moist with a plastic overwrap.

The onion poultices may be kept on overnight, and repeated several nights in a row. This accelerates healing.

STRAIN

A strain is an injury resulting from excessive use of the body.

Water Therapy

Apply cold water compresses, firm dressing, and either elevate or immobilize the injured area.

General Therapy

In addition to immobilization, adhesive strapping may be necessary.

BUNION

Water Therapy

Add alum powder to warm foot bath, and soak the afflicted foot. Whirlpool therapy will increase the circulation. Dry and cool bunion area.

General Therapy

A bunion is a swelling of the bursa of the toe or foot joint. It always helps to restore the toe to a *normal position*. To do this, tape along the toe with a 1-inch strip of adhesive, and gently pull toe into normal position. Repeat periodically.

BURNS

There are several excellent home remedies for minor burns, but cold or ice water is always the preferred initial treatment. The use of cold and/or ice water was reinstated by physicians after World War II. During the "Russian Run," there were hundreds of severely burned torpedo victims. Many of the burned merchant marine *survivors* were those who had been completely immersed in the icy arctic water.

Water Therapy

Depending on the burn, immerse the burned area in cold running water. This is usually all you will need for such minor mishaps as touching a hot pot or a hot iron. You may also immerse in ice water or possibly apply ice water compresses (not for bad burns, as the cloth might stick).

General Therapy

After the ice cold water treatment, you can also apply these effective home remedies:

1. Vitamin E oil or ointment (or open a capsule).

2. Juice from inside the leaf of an aloe plant. These are very easy to grow as house plants. They thrive with very little watering.

3. PABA ointment or cream. PABA is one of the B vitamins, is very useful for burns, and is also an excellent internal and external remedy for light-skinned people who are sensitive to sunburn.

4. For throbbing pain, in addition to ice and one of the above remedies, wrapping the burn area in clay, and keeping out the air, can contain the pain.

For serious burns, rush the patient to a hospital or burn center.

BUTTOCKS
(strawberry bruise)

Water Therapy

A strawberry is a superficial abrasion of the skin that commonly occurs to sliding base runners. Immediately cleanse the strawberry with soap and warm water. This may smart. Calendula or chamomile tea may be used instead of soap and water for a more soothing effect.

General Therapy

Apply a nonsensitizing ointment such as calendula or comfrey to quickly heal the abrasion.

CALLUS

Water Therapy

Build-up of hardened tissue on the soles or the heels can interfere with normal or, especially, athletic activity. Prevent this build-up or soften the tissue by taking hot epsom salt foot baths.

General Therapy

In addition to the foot baths, file the area with a special callus file. Do *not* hone the area with a razor blade. To maintain a soft and pliable foot, also rub a lanolin-based ointment into the callus and potential callus areas. Place a thin moleskin pad over the callus, and attach with tape.

SWIMMER'S CALLUS

Water Therapy

Heal the cracked callus with herbal ointments (see below). Then, harden the feet with frequent foot baths of cold to tepid water and alum, and also by treading in cold water. Increase foot circulation with alternate hot and cold showers.

General Therapy

Bleeding may occur in the edges of deep cracks along the edge of the feet because the water leeches out the natural oils of the body. Apply calendula ointment to heal the cracks.

CALF CRAMPS

Water Therapy

Many people have painful nighttime cramps. Hot whirlpool baths will relieve the problem temporarily. However, any other local heat applications or ice may bring on additional spasms. It greatly helps to knead any knots before, during, and after the whirlpool baths.

When the cramps are due mainly to athletic or dance activity, it may be because the body has a depletion of water and salt. Add a small amount of salt to your drinking water, or take several salt tablets before performances, practice, or competition. Salt must be flushed down with lots of water.

Also drink lots of water before, during, and after all athletic or dance activities.

General Therapy

Increase the calcium and vitamin C intake. Eat foods high in potassium.

CHAFING

Water Therapy

To overcome a chafing irritation on the inside of the thighs or the buttocks, apply a paste of colloidal or finely blended cooking oatmeal or corn starch to the area, and soak in a long warm oatmeal or cornstarch bath.

To both strengthen the body and regulate skin activity, take frequent cold water baths. Children susceptible to chafing should be briefly dipped into cold water 3 times a day. This will gradually overcome the problem, and also greatly increase vitality and stamina.

General Therapy

Wear cotton underpants to absorb perspiration. The area of chafing needs washing, lubrication (use calendula ointment) and powdering (use corn starch or baby powder) each day. If the chafing occurs during athletic activity, males should add absorbent cotton inside the athletic support.

CHAPPED SKIN

Water Therapy

Apply a warm compress that has been dipped in hayflower tea to chapped area once a day. In addition, plunge arms and/or feet into cold water once a day for 4–5 minutes. This procedure works for children as well.

General Therapy

There are many soothing natural substances that heal the skin. Use either the juice from an aloe leaf, vitamin E oil, calendula ointment, or glycerine and rose water.

CHEST INJURIES
(see also Bronchitis, Coughing, Congestion)

CHEST CONGESTION
Water Therapy

The object of the water therapy is to divert the congestion in the chest. Take either a hot leg bath, or alternate hot and cold footbaths. You can also release the congestion by using mild mustard, cayenne, or ginger powder packs.

CHEST STRAIN (PECTORAL STRAIN)

Water Therapy

A wild swing with a heavy object or too many pushups can create a chest strain. Besides feeling sore, there may also be swelling. This indicates some muscle fiber separation and bleeding.

If the area remains swollen for 24–48 hours, apply ice to the area of pain in 20-minute segments. Do this every six hours for one day.

General Therapy

Apply a sling to the arm on the side of the strain. If the strain occurs on both sides, suspend all activity that is even remotely strenuous. Symptoms tend to disappear within a few days unless there is swelling, in which case recovery may take about a week. Do not force movement. This injury must be allowed to heal *naturally*. Do not use pain killers. Because they mask the pain, they may cause a permanently torn pectoral muscle.

FLOATING RIBS

Water Therapy

Our ribs are constantly moving, but in young people the eleventh and twelfth ribs actually "float." A sharp impact to these two ribs results in swelling and pain, and causes difficulty in walking.

Ice therapy, used several times a day in 30-minute segments, will numb the initial pain and control swelling and possible internal bleeding.

General Therapy

This kind of injury usually occurs during athletic competition. The athlete must check with a physician, and participate in a program of systematic and gradual exercises for a week before returning to competition.

CHICKEN POX
(see also Scarlet Fever, Measles)

Water Therapy

For a mild case of chicken pox, flush the system with copious quantities of drinking water and several rectal irrigations. Use the dry hot blanket pack to induce perspiration.

Several times a day when the temperature is high, take 20–30 minute tepid baths (about 90°F). Also, if there is even a slight fever, apply a cold abdominal compress every half hour. Renew whenever the compress is warm and dry.

For a more difficult case of chicken pox, follow the instructions for measles or scarlet fever.

CHILBLAINS
(see also Frostbite)

Chilblains is a localized, recurrent itching, swelling, and pain, and redness on fingers, toes, and ears, produced by a mild frostbite.

Water Therapy

Use either short cold foot baths, or alternate, *equal* 15-second hot and cold showers to the area of pain.

CHILDBIRTH
(see also Pregnancy)

Water Therapy

Drink copious quantities of red raspberry leaf tea before, during, and after giving birth. This tea helps to overcome many bleeding problems and also alleviates thirst.

If the birth is to take place at home: Short or prolonged cold compresses to the breasts or showers directed to the breasts can, when needed, cause vigorous contractions of the uterus.

Short cold foot baths also act via reflex on the abdominal, pelvic, and head regions, stimulating them and increasing circulation. This causes contractions in the uterus.

Do not use these foot baths in the early stages of pregnancy.

To relax the uterine tissues while giving birth, apply hot moist compresses over the pubic area, and the area between the vagina and anus.

In the early stages of labor, to mollify pain and promote relaxation, take a warm deep sit bath.

Two days after delivery, a hot dry pack can be applied to the breasts to encourage perspiration and help bring on the milk. Also, hot apple cider vinegar and water douches can be used to soothe the vaginal area.

After the 5th day, a cold sheet pack may be placed over the abdomen and breasts to prevent any possible congestion, and to lessen the possibility of the nipples cracking and caking. (Also see Breasts: page 121)

You can feed the infant a teaspoon of *pure* room-temperature water before breast feeding. This dilutes the milk, promotes emulsion of fats, and supplies the baby with additional mineral salts.

CHRONIC DISEASES

With any chronic problem, it is imperative to stimulate the skin, as this will encourage the release of toxins by perspiration or elimination. It is imperative that the pores of the skin always be open. If they were to become entirely closed, the skin could no longer breathe and we would die.

Water Therapy

As often as possible follow any or all of these procedures:
1. Dry brush massage with wash cloth or natural bristle brush.
2. Frequent soapings of the entire body.

3. Frequent shampoos to stimulate the scalp. Use an organic or herbal soap. Rinse the hair with diluted apple cider vinegar to restore the acid mantle of the hair and eliminate soap residue.

4. On arising, pull, rub, and stretch the fingers and toes. Follow this with a brief cold water tread. Then soap the body and take a long warm shower. Use a rough wash cloth to remove dry skin cells. To tone and vitalize the body, conclude with a brief cool shower.

5. Once a week use a perspiration-inducing technique such as:

a. Damp sheet compress (half or three-quarter compress can be used)

b. Hot hayflower or hot epsom salt bath (cold compress on forehead)

c. Oil bath. Oil body with a mixture of equal parts deodorized castor oil and olive oil. Wait 15 minutes. Soak in a moderately hot bath, and brush the skin.

After bath or compress, go to bed to perspire. Remain in bed for one to several hours. Then take a warm shower and soap off any sludgy waste that has been exuded. Conclude shower with a cool water splash. Eventually work up to a cold water splash. Pat diluted or full-strength apple cider vinegar over the body, except near eyes and genitals. This restores the acid mantle of the skin. End with another brief cold water foot bath.

General Therapy

Practice two 20-minute mental imagery sessions.

The following sequence has been very successful in overcoming many disease states. It helps to relax the body, marshal antibodies, and increase healing life-force energy.

1. Mentally relax every inch of your body. Start with the top of the head, and item by item work down to the toes. If any area is still tense, go back and mentally and physically relax that part. Often you will find that jaws or eyes or neck are extremely tense. But each person has personal vulnerable areas.

2. Prepare to take a mental "trip."

a. Count backward from 10 to 1, and concentrate on a way of "moving *down.*" Some people walk down stairs, a mountain, or take an elevator or escalator.

b. Visualize the *most beautiful* place you have ever seen. It can be a place you have visited and vowed to return to, or a scene from a movie, or a photograph. Perhaps it is a beach and a cove, or a pine forest, or a mountain view over a valley, or a river stream. This is *your place* to return to. Whenever you are stressed, you will return *instantly* to this spot, and you will feel *regenerated.*

c. Breathe deeply and rhythmically. Imagine the *texture* of flowers, leaves, sand, or water. *Smell* the air. *Listen* for the sounds. Is the water making a lapping sound? Are the birds singing? Is there wind through leaves? Be quiet and enjoy your visit. If you wish, you can imagine walking, running, or swimming there. See your-self *smiling, happy,* and *carefree.*

d. After 10 minutes of this mental "vacation" count forward from 1 to 10, come "back," *smile,* and next:

e. Imagine a *huge balloon of white light.* If you prefer another heal-ing color, change the color. Concentrate this white light balloon on the damaged, diseased, or injured part of the body. Mobilize millions of *useful white blood corpuscles,* and march them in like an army to take over and overcome any chronic disease. In your mind, see these white corpuscles sizzling through the inflamma-tion, painful area, or diseased portion of your body.

f. In your mind, "see" that area or areas of the body completely healed.

Remember always that the *desire to be well* and the *confidence that you will be well* are important aids in achieving a healthy state. This type of sequence is useful for limited pain injuries, as well as so-called terminal cases, many of which have shown astonishing improvement by this inter-nal mobilization of healing forces.

CIRCULATION

Water Therapy

Circulation is one of the keys to good health. One of the foremost circulation boosters is cold water. All cold water treatments are energiz-ing, and after you use them for a while, with increasingly colder and colder water, you'll feel remarkably stronger.

The following are the best cold, and cold and friction, procedures. All will increase circulation patterns.

1. Treading in cold water. Walk in cold water up to the ankles or calves. An adjunct to this therapy is to walk in wet grass, on wet pebbles, or in snow.

2. Cold friction massage. This is achieved by sectional friction rub-bing with cold water. This is the preferred washing technique for persons weakened by fever, age, or chronic disease.

3. Salt massage. Rub the body with a paste of common salt before taking a warm shower or warm bath. Conclude the shower or bath with cool water splash.

4. Partial cold showers directed to one area at a time will provide long-term circulation benefits.

5. Ginger baths will aid circulation. Add a small amount of pow-dered ginger or ginger root tea to the warm bath. End the bath with cool splashes on the feet and the entire body. This is quite stimulating for the body.

6. Rosemary tea, or professional rosemary bath extracts or lotions, are stimulating for the skin and increase circulation. Rosemary is one of the ingredients in the famed Queen of Hungary Water, used as a stimulat-ing liniment for injured or paralyzed limbs.

CLEAT BRUISES

Water Therapy

If there is no fracture, apply a wrapped ice bag to bruise and attach with an elastic bandage. Elevate the area. This usually solves the problem within a day.

General Therapy

There will be extreme tenderness in the area. To prevent further impact, use rubber padding on the area for about 2 weeks. Apply a healing ointment such as calendula.

COLDS

Water Therapy

Drink copious amounts of water to flush out the system. Use baths and friction massages to help eliminate stored toxins and to reenergize the body.

An ice cube massage on the *large toes* increases circulation in the body.

All tonic friction methods will increase the elimination of toxins and help to overcome energy blocks.

Drink copious quantities of pure water and/or herbal teas. Hot herbal teas before, during, and after any detoxification bath will increase perspiration. Peppermint and sage are my favorites. I add a tiny pinch of cayenne pepper for the digestive system, and a tiny pinch of ginseng powder to stabilize the rest of the system and increase energy. Ginseng is helpful for chest complaints too. To increase perspiration, combine larger amounts of peppermint with smaller amounts of yarrow and elderflower, or a pinch of boneset. Add honey to sweeten. If the digestive system is "off," be sure to use the cayenne pepper. Cloves, caraway, and anise may also be added.

As soon as you feel you are coming down with a cold, take a detoxifying bath such as hayflower, oatstraw, epsom salt, pine, or sage. Start the bath with an invigorating salt rub or apple cider vinegar splash. Use a wash cloth, brush, or loofah to stimulate skin action and elimination through perspiration. Return to bed for a one-hour perspiration session, or for a long restful sleep. If you prefer, you may first wash off the body with warm water. Splash cold water on the ankles or take a very brief cold foot bath to stimulate the body. Again, splash the apple cider vinegar on the body, as this lessens fatigue and restores an acid mantle barrier.

If you have a sore throat, also apply a cold, or apple cider vinegar, double throat compress or larger triangular compress.

COLD FEET AND COLD HANDS

Cold feet and cold hands are a problem of general circulation.

Water Therapy

Direct a cold jet shower to the soles of the feet.

Walk each day, several times a day if possible, in cold water up to the calves, or splash cold water over the ankles in the morning and before bedtime.

Apply a cold compress to the *back* of the neck, and sit briefly in a cold shallow bath.

Use rosemary oil, or rosemary bath lotion, in the bath. Also add a few grains of cayenne pepper in one hot herbal drink each day. This will help digestion and aid internal circulation.

COLD BODY

Water Therapy

When the body has lost heat, it is necessary to rebalance the heat mechanism. There are several excellent water therapy procedures which will accomplish this.

The best procedure for the severe loss of body heat is the dry blanket pack. Add a few hot water bottles (or hot water in tightly lidded jars) to quickly warm up the body.

Other excellent water therapies are immersion in a warm bath; drinking hot, stimulating herbal preparations such as peppermint tea with a pinch of cayenne pepper; or massaging the body with sectional cold-water friction methods.

General Therapy

If you are *outdoors,* make sure your head and hands are covered, as otherwise there is a sharp reduction of body heat. *Move around.* Try not to sweat. Keep *cool* instead of hot when working. Never drink alcohol when the weather is extremely cold. Keep your feet as dry as possible.

COLIC

Water Therapy

A hot shallow sit bath or a hot foot bath will help to overcome stomach spasms by reflex action.

Chamomile is a very effective remedy for controlling colic in children. Make a tea by adding boiling water to the flowers. Steep, cool, and strain into a cup or a baby's bottle. It relieves stomach upsets and spasms.

General Therapy

When in doubt about severe and persistent gas pains, see a physician.

COLITIS
(see also Digestive Problems, Constipation)

Water Therapy

Spasm: Apply a hot moist compress to abdomen.
Gas: Apply a cold wet pack to abdomen, cover with dry towel, and cover the entire body with warm bedclothes.

To remove excess mucus: Take a honey and salt enema in a knee-chest position, and retain water as long as 20 minutes. This will bring down much of the mucus, but *it will be painful.* To help remove the pain, apply a hot moist compress on abdomen during the enema.

Afterward, relieve the weakness in the body by washing with a cold friction rub.

Take the enema 3 times a week, and continue up to 6 weeks or until there is little or no mucus brought away by the salt solution. Then follow a simultaneous therapy of hot compresses to the abdomen and hot foot baths. Conclude the treatment with a cold friction massage.

Each day before dinner, take a general massage to tone the body; rub the spine by lying on a rolled up towel; or use alternate hot and very short cold (Scots) showers directed to the spine.

General Therapy

Colitis is a situation that demands holistic thinking. Determine the *cause* of the attacks. They may stem from stress, allergies, inability to digest roughage, or imbalance due to antibiotics. To offset antibiotic intake, eat kefir or yogurt, or take acidophilus tablets each day.

Fasting for a week on a vegetable juice, or following a one item (mono) diet, and only eating many *small* meals, chewing thoroughly and *slowly,* can help the healing process. The following food items will help natural healing:

1. Bananas.
2. Eat raw salads—alfalfa, mung, and lentil sprouts are good—but eat the vegetables very slowly and thoroughly.
3. Two tablespoons of olive oil or any other cold-pressed oil each day.
4. Raw cabbage juice.
5. Kamillosan liquid, an extract of chamomile for internal and external use, is available from Weleda. Add several drops to tea.
6. Enzyme tablets such as papaya or pepsin, added to the diet.

Do not eat too many carbohydrates, except cooked millet.

CONGESTION

Water Therapy

Alternate hot and cold partial baths, showers, or compresses directed to the limbs will relieve congestion in acute or chronic problems.

The alternate applications work in this way: As the temperature changes from hot to cold, it creates a widening and narrowing of the

LESSEN INFLAMMATION BY DEPLETION ACTION

A *depletion action* lessens the amount of blood in a given part of the body. This technique is useful in relieving congestion and inflammation.

Deplete Area of Inflammation	Apply Water Here
SCIATICA	Large *hot moist compresses* to back and side of thigh, to divert the blood from the nerves of the skin.
TRIGEMINAL NEURALGIA	*Hot moist heat* to side of face. This immediately diverts the blood to the skin. This can be reinforced by *ice bag* over carotid artery, as this mechanically lessens the volume of blood to the head. Do not use cold *over* the seat of the pain, as it will increase this pain.
APPENDICITIS	Hot *hip and leg pack* and *ice bag* over the appendix.
MENINGITIS	*Hot leg pack*, with *ice bags* to base of brain and upper spine.
PERITONITIS	*Hot hip and leg pack*, or *leg pack* only. *Ice compress* or *ice bag* to abdomen.
BOIL	Early stage of the boil can be aborted by applying an *ice bag* directly over the seat of the infection.

blood vessels. This quickly increases the white blood cells in the congested part. This is very helpful in cases of infection and inflammation in the hand or foot. In addition, the constriction and dilation of the blood vessels encourage circulation of the blood. This helps in the long-range treatment of chronic congestion.

See specific instructions for each problem, and charts on pages 170–171.

CONSTIPATION

Water Therapy

Drinking: One of the very best answers to many chronic cases of constipation is a simple one: drink 2 glasses of *cold* water on arising. Try to wait about 1 hour before eating breakfast. The early cleansing drink stimulates gastric secretions. I drink Mountain Valley water.

Continue to drink either pure water, or fruit juices, or herbal drinks during the day. It helps if you can drink about 8 glasses of water.

Showers: Contrast showers of long hot and short cold streams, directed to the abdomen, and an occasional shower directed to the anal area, tone the digestive and eliminative organs.

Long term digestive problems are well served with the cold abdominal compress (or pack). This cold wrapping, covered with a larger, dry overwrapping, may be worn to bed. When used for months, this compress greatly tones the digestive and eliminative organs.

Reflex water therapy includes using hot shoulder shower, cold hip spray shower, cold back shower, or occasional spray over the entire body. Occasional cold half baths of a few seconds are stimulating.

For *spastic constipation*, take hot enemas, and drink copious amounts of chamomile tea.

Feed *constipated children* a teaspoon of cold water every hour. Several times during the week briefly dip the child into cold baths up to the armpits.

General Therapy

If nothing else works, try hydrochloride and pepsin, or hydrochloride and betaine tablets. Eat these with meals. Many people have a depleted hydrochloric acid production, and need additional supplements with one or all meals. Sometimes this therapy can be effective in only a short time, but it may also be a lifetime need.

Do not, however, take any of these tablets if you have a peptic or stomach ulcer.

CONTUSION
(see Bruises)

CONVULSIONS
(Children)

Water Therapy

Use the *warm pack*, or a modified cold wrap. Place a long cotton nightgown on the child. Dip the child and nightgown briefly into cold water in the bathtub, and then quickly wrap the child in an old flannel or wool blanket. Place the child in bed and cover him with a light blanket or feather cover. Repeat procedure several times if necessary.

COUGHING
(see also Bronchitis)

Water Therapy

Breathe in steam to which a teaspoon of tincture of benzoin has been added. Massage the sides, back, and front of neck with ice in a clockwise fashion. Immediately follow ice massage with hot and moist compresses to the same area.

A cold wet double compress on the chest will act in a stimulating fashion. When renewed every 30 minutes it modifies the cough, eases expectoration, relieves labored breathing, improves chest circulation, and improves general circulation.

CRYING SPELLS
(Children)

Water Therapy

First try adding linden or chamomile tea to the drinking water or bottle. This will help to overcome spasms and trapped gas. If there doesn't seem to be a reason for the crying, apply the wet cold abdominal compress, and cover with a flannel blanket. This technique is highly successful. Repeat twice a day until the crying spells stop.

General Therapy

The water remedies work either to alleviate spasms, or totally alter body imbalance. You can also use the Bach Flower Remedies. See Resource List. Place 2 drops of Bach walnut flowers or 2 drops of Bach chicory flowers in a small amount of water. Have the child drink the preparation. These nontoxic flower infusions will also work on tearful adults.

CYSTITIS

Cystitis is an inflammation or infection in the bladder. This usually occurs as a result of infections of associated organs: kidney, prostate, urethra. It may be acute or chronic.

Water Therapy

Acute attacks: (Use *only* hot treatments)

Take hot shallow sit baths several times a day.

Take hot footbaths several times a day.

Add hot catnip tea to enema to relieve spasm or constipation.

General Therapy

To prevent yeast infection, take capsules of acidophilus every day. Add solution of acidophilus to *vaginal douche.*

Drink 2 glasses of cranberry juice every day.

Drink apple cider vinegar, honey, and water mixed. Add 1 tablespoon of vinegar and honey each to every cup of hot or cold water. This helps to establish internal balance.

Eat large amounts of *watermelon.* Cut the red flesh into tiny pieces, and eat one piece every 10 minutes or so throughout the day. This will flush the kidneys and bladder.

Add vitamin C to the diet and drink vegetable juices. Add small amounts of parsley or corn silk tea to peppermint or chamomile tea; or make parsley soup. Other herbs that are helpful in cystitis are juniper berries, golden rod (tea), and horsetail (tea).

DIABETES

Water Therapy

Drinking water decreases the amount of sugar in the system. Drink several quarts of hot water (you can use hot herbal teas) *between meals.* It is important to drink hard water with a high mineral content.

Cold showers increase oxidation more than 100% according to tests on diabetic patients. This is valuable to diabetics because it prevents some of the secondary skin problems associated with this disease, and releases the unoxidized sugar through the skin and the kidneys.

Take cold showers with pressure percussion spray. Follow with cold friction massage.

Occasionally use alternate long hot and short cold (Scots) showers. Always conclude with a cold shower.

Apply a cold abdominal compress to give long-term stimulus to digestive and other organs.

General Therapy

Exercise is vital for the diabetic, particularly to overcome their susceptibility to fatigue. Both Swedish massage and swimming give good results. Dancer Allegra Kent's *Water Beauty Book* offers excellent water exercises.

DIARRHEA

Water Therapy

Acute attack: An unusual flow of wastes (diarrhea) from the body is the natural way the body eliminates toxins from the body in an acute bacterial or parasitic attack. However, if and when the diarrhea is so severe that it becomes a menace to recovery, you must stop it. The goal of the water therapy is to help the body to eliminate the poisons causing the attack. *Stop eating* during the attack.

To help in elimination, use an enema. This may seem strange considering the nature of the problem, but it flushes out the colon, and is most helpful. Repeated hot rectal irrigations cause the kidney to function when even drugs fail. Repeat every half hour if necessary. In the case of food poisoning, use a pure, undiluted, hot coffee enema, as it is detoxifying.

If a child has a severe attack of diarrhea, flush the anal area with cold sterile water after each bowel movement.

Take cold baths with either hayflower or apple cider vinegar. This allows some toxins to be eliminated through the skin.

Apply cold double apple cider vinegar compresses to the abdomen. These have a heating effect. Drink hot herbal teas, and sponge the body with cold water or diluted apple cider vinegar or hayflower tea. Repeat sponging every 3 hours.

To stop diarrhea: If it is an emergency, you can stop the flow of waste material by sitting in a cold shallow bath, 40°F–50°F, for 10 minutes. While in the bath, massage the body vigorously. Dry the body with intense friction rubbing.

To control pain and reduce vomiting: You can inhibit pain and vomiting somewhat by placing a hot apple cider vinegar and water compress on the abdomen. If there is severe diarrhea, also apply an abdominal bandage.

Children (chronic attacks): Strengthen the child's system and eliminate the diarrhea attacks with these two water therapy applications:

1. Cold half baths for a few seconds every day for the first week. Afterward, use every other day.

2. For one to several weeks afterward, apply a cold abdominal compress. Use either cold or warm water, or diluted apple cider vinegar. Use

a fresh compress every day. This will absorb diseased toxins from the system and tone up the internal organs.

When in doubt about persistent diarrhea, see your physician.

General Therapy

Stop eating, or go on a mono diet. Eat cooked, peeled apples, or peeled, diced apples (pectin-rich), or lots of white rice, to bind and cleanse the body.

Acidophilus tablets or yogurt will help to restore the natural intestinal flora.

For children, make a soup made of either cooked carrots *(excellent)* or barley to restore the water level and control the diarrhea. Bananas and buttermilk are also beneficial.

Dried blueberries or blueberry extract, extract of peppermint, chamomile tea, peppermint tea, witch hazel leaf tea, or raspberry leaf tea, activated charcoal or clay water are all excellent. A few grains of cayenne in water or tea often stops the queasiness.

After the situation clears up, drink papaya juice or lemon juice or fresh pineapple juice to restore flushed out enzymes.

DIGESTIVE PROBLEMS

FLATULENCE

Water Therapy

Direct a cold, no-pressure fan shower to the area below the ribs to the navel. As often as possible take brief cold shallow sit baths. Drink peppermint, chamomile, or rosemary tea. Add a pinch of bruised anise or caraway seed if desired.

General Therapy

Rub the abdomen in clockwise fashion.

Eat food slowly and thoroughly. Provide a restful atmosphere at meals.

STOMACH WEAKNESS

Water Therapy

To increase the muscular action of the stomach, direct a cold, no-pressure fan spray over midline stomach area below the ribs to the navel.

General Therapy

Drink rosemary tea before and after each meal. It may be sweetened with honey. Rosemary helps to activate the liver and enzymes.

STOMACH SPASMS

Water Therapy

For stomach spasms or ulcer pain or duodenal catarrh, direct a hot, "broken," weak pressure, fan-shaped shower to midline stomach area below the ribs to the navel.

Drink linden or chamomile tea. An excellent chamomile extract, Kamillosan liquid, is available through Weleda.

EXCESS GASTRIC ACIDITY

Water Therapy

A 10-minute hot water epsom salt bath (using 1½ pounds of the salts) will neutralize accumulated acid wastes in the body.

Do not do this if you have a heart problem.

As often as possible wear a double cold abdominal compress, or apply a cold wet towel over the abdomen, and cover with a dry towel. This has a heating effect and will tone the digestive organs. Change the compress when it becomes warm, or wear it during sleep.

VOMITING

Water Therapy

Apply one ice bag over the stomach, and another between the shoulders.

PAIN

Water Therapy

Apply a hot moist compress *between the shoulders.* Add a hot water bottle over the compress to retain the heat for a longer time. *At the same time,* apply a hot moist compress, covered with dry cloth, to the *abdomen.* Renew every 10 minutes.

FOOD POISONING

Water Therapy

Drink lukewarm water. This simple measure is often effective in bringing up the toxic material. If needed, add a pinch of mustard powder or a pinch of salt to the tepid water as an emetic.

Irrigate the colon with an enema of nondiluted, nondecaffeinated coffee. This quickly detoxifies the body and relieves natural pain and pressure. Sometimes this enema quickens the vomiting process.

INFLAMMATION OF STOMACH LINING

Water Therapy

Note above details on pain and vomiting.

Immerse body in alternate hot and cold hip baths, and conclude with a cold sponging of the entire body. Another excellent therapy is a very hot (115°F) low-pressure, fan-type shower directed to the area below the ribs to the navel. This stimulates the muscular action of the stomach, as well as Meisner's and Auerbach's plexus.

CHRONIC GASTRITIS

Water Therapy

Sip 2 glasses of *hot* water every morning before breakfast.

Take a 10-minute warm bath first thing each morning. Conclude the bath with a cold shower and a vigorous towel rub.

Apply a cold abdominal compress before going to sleep. You can either remove it when it gets warm, or leave it on all night. The compress stimulates the digestive organs.

LACK OF GASTRIC JUICE

Water Therapy

Drink a large glass of ice water *before meals.* Do not drink any other fluid *with* the meals. The ice water stimulates the gastric glands in the stomach, and the flow of the digestive juices.

Ten minutes before bedtime, apply a cold wet towel to the abdomen. Cover this with a dry towel. Cover the entire body with bedcovers.

DYSPEPSIA

Water Therapy

An alternate long hot and short cold (Scots) shower with pressure, applied at the midline under the ribs to the navel, will relieve dyspepsia. This same shower will help intercostal pain due to neuralgia, and pain between the shoulders.

General Therapy (All Digestive Problems)

Indigestion and flatulence are usually due to poorly digested proteins and carbohydrates, or the lack of, or too much, gastric juice. Since many people over 40, and still more over 50 and 65, have only a portion of the hydrochloric acid they need in their systems, it is often necessary to add hydrochloric acid with betaine or pepsin after each meal. This may help cure constipation, as the HCL effects elimination of all digestive waste products.

Anyone with a peptic or stomach ulcer should not take HCL.

Eating only one food at each meal (a mono diet) can be a help in overcoming some digestive problems, and frequent fasts of one juice only will rest the digestive organs.

Drink rosemary tea to cleanse the liver. Drink chamomile tea and peppermint tea for most digestive problems, especially spasms and diarrhea. For flatulence, add the strained juice of bruised anise, fennel, or caraway seeds.

DIPHTHERIA

The following water therapies were used by physician hydrotherapists before the creation of antibiotics. If there is an outbreak of this disease, use these therapies until your physician can be reached.

Water Therapy

Snugly wrap the child's neck in a damp cold water compress, or diluted apple cider vinegar compress. Replace as soon as it is hot, every 15 minutes or so. For body wrapping, use a long cotton nightgown or two pinned hand towels, or bath towels. Dip the towels or nightgown into a mixture of half apple cider vinegar and half water, wring out so that it is still damp, and wrap it around the child from his or her *armpits to knees.* Pin. Cover child with bedclothes. Change wrapping every 15 minutes until the body heat decreases. The child should also drink copious amounts of water and pineapple juice. The latter seems to be helpful in detaching the membrane on the throat.

Several times a day: Flush out colon with enema. Use a vaporizer in the room with pineapple juice in the water. Use cold sectional sponging every 3-4 hours to stimulate the nervous system and the heart. If there is numbness in the body, apply a hot moist compress on the affected nerves for 20 minutes. Follow each hot application with a cold sponging and swift drying of the area. Do not allow drafts.

Between treatments: Apply a cold compress to the heart area. This acts as a tonic.

Threat of suffocation: Place the child in full hot bath for 1 to 20 minutes. At the same time use cold water to sponge the back of the neck, the entire back, the shoulders, and spine area.

Dr. Kuhn of Germany has experimented with an ice water spray over the membrane of the throat. This helps to loosen the membrane. If the patient cooperates and *expectorates as soon as the water touches the throat, the throat can be cleared.* Repeat every half hour.

DIURETICS

Water Therapy

Water therapies can promote perspiration which releases stored liquids, or stimulate the kidneys to release the liquid through urine.

Drink one of the several bottled waters on the market that act as a natural diuretic. Mountain Valley Water is one such pure water. If this is not possible, drink plain water.

Also drink parsley tea, or corn silk tea, or eat watermelon, as these flush the system and kidneys.

To promote additional release of fluids, apply any or all of these therapies: hot moist compresses to lower back; cold spray directed to lower breast bone and lower back; alternate long hot and short cold spray on lower breastbone and lower back.

The following water therapies increase the release of fluids through perspiration: full blanket pack, partial blanket pack, sauna, Russian or Turkish baths, cold trunk pack.

General Therapy (Chemical Diuretics and Sports)

Sometimes wrestlers are urged to lose weight prior to the match in order to compete in a lighter weight class. This may lead to long-term problems, as well as acute mineral loss. Sports physicians urge young athletes to think about whether you want to please the coach or please your *own body.*

DIZZINESS
(Children)
Water Therapy

Dizziness *may* be due to sluggishness of the liver. The liver may be stimulated with occasional enemas. The child should drink 2 glasses of cold water a half hour before breakfast.

Apply a towel dipped in half apple cider vinegar and half cold water, and wind around the child from the armpits to the knees, several times a day for 1 hour at a time.

DRUNKENNESS
Water Therapy

A drunken person can be aroused from a stupor by a dousing or by having water applied from a height. You can do this by throwing a pail of cold water at the person or putting him under a cold shower. Fast cold friction sponging will also arouse the person. It is imperative to *friction rub the body* with a towel after dousing, to prevent complications.

EAR PROBLEMS
(see also page 56)
GENERAL

Water Therapy

In general, hot moist compresses are helpful for inflammations of the outer ear structures. This includes some abscesses. Alternate hot and cold applications can increase the absorption of inflammatory deposits. A warm baby's syringe spray removes hardened ear wax, foreign objects, and insects.

Two other applications are very helpful with ear problems. Apply a double throat compress made either with cold water or cold water mixed with apple cider vinegar, or use both the throat and *ear windings.*

Foot wrappings, compresses, or foot baths stimulate blood flow in the feet and divert the blood flow away from a congested ear.

General Therapy

To relieve pain in the ear, place a small piece of cotton that has been drenched in warm mullein (see Resource List) or almond oil in the ear. In an emergency, use hot olive, corn, or safflower oil.

Hot salt bags are excellent aids in relieving acute ear pain. Place about 2 pounds of coarse salt in a cotton pillow case or towel. Close with safety pins. Place the salt bag in a container and heat it in a slow oven until the bag is hot. Place this in still another small pillow case (to contain the heat) and apply to ear. The hot salt will relieve the pain, and draw out any pus in the ear.

If salt is not available, heat up the inside of a rye or white bread, and pound in bruised caraway seeds. This will also draw out the pain.

To remove wax, dip a cotton swab into hot oil and gently cleanse the ear. Hot oil applications also help relieve cramps in the ear, and overcome some ear humming problems. After placing drops in ear, plug the ear with cotton.

Children

Ear infections in children may be an allergic reaction—probably adrenal gland exhaustion. Vitamin C and pantothenic acid (a B vitamin) are needed to produce natural cortisone to stimulate the adrenal glands. It is a good idea to eliminate milk from the child's diet, although raw milk and ice cream are okay. The child should be encouraged to eat many small meals a day, and should be given seven 500-milligram doses of vitamin C and a big dose of vitamin B daily.

You should consult your child's pediatricain about this regimen.

INFLAMMATION OF MIDDLE EAR (Otitis Media)

This middle ear infection can follow in the wake of measles, mumps, pneumonia, influenza, or scarlet fever.

Water Therapy

Relieve pain by warm treatments. Apply a *dry,* wrapped hot water bottle to ear.

For severe pain, apply moist hot compresses on ear, and *simultaneously* apply an ice bag, or frozen bandage, just below the jaw of the painful ear. The cold application contracts the large vessels of the neck and diminishes the pain in the area. Heated almond oil or heated mullein oil may be added to the hot compress cloth.

INFLAMMATION OF LINING OF EAR CANAL (Otitis Externa)

Because the taut shape of the ear does not allow tissue to swell, what might well be a mild and localized inflammation in another part of the body becomes in the ear a painful and widespread infection, otitis externa. This infection sometimes results from swimming, and is a condition often seen in competitive swimming.

Water Therapy

Dilute Burrow's Solution to half strength with water, and gently cleanse the outer ear passage. Dry the ears gently, and do not scratch!

Relieve the pain with warmth. Apply a dry, wrapped hot water bottle or a moist, hot compress to the ear.

General Therapy

Stay out of the pool until there is a full recovery.

ECZEMA

Water Therapy

Children: Children with eczema respond to a program of hayflower wrappings, or hayflower-dipped shirts. The "compress" absorbs the diseased material from the body. Repeat this 3 times a week for 3 months.

Once a week wash the child's head with warm horsetail tea.

General toning applications: Since eczema is a stress reaction and a chronic condition, it is important to strengthen the body with frequent neutral half baths, cold spongings, and alternate hot and cold showers directed to the thigh and upper chest.

Wet eczema responds to most cold water strengthening treatments, particularly those directed to the stomach area and those that affect digestion.

General Therapy

Eczema is such a variable problem that you must experiment with the general treatments to find which ones work the best for you. Oatmeal soaps and colloidal oatmeal washes are often helpful. Applications of vitamin E oil can help overcome the dryness. Napier's (Edinburgh) "Slippery Elm" soap helps some people, and Nelson's (London) "Calendula and Hamamelis Hand and Skin Lotion" has also been used successfully.

Eczema patients may occasionally use valerian discotes to calm the nerves. The Bach Flower Remedies, which help change your emotional state, are also effective.

Many persons who suffer from eczema need an additional intake of vegetable oils and/or vitamin F.

ELIMINATION
(see also Bladder, Chronic Diseases, Eruptions,
Kidney Problems, and Perspiration)

Water Therapy

A long hot bath will help to induce perspiration through the pores of the skin.

An enema will aid in evacuation of retained wastes.

A mono diet as well as juice fasts will stimulate elimination of wastes through the pores.

Hot hayflower or oatstraw baths help detoxify the body.

A coffee enema will remove any poisoned food from the body, and help detoxify the body during chronic disease.

ERUPTIONS
CHILDREN (see also Chicken Pox, Measles, Scarlet Fever)

Water Therapy

Bacterial infections: If there is a threat of a scarlet fever or measles epidemic, or any bacterial epidemic, bring out the eruptions and toxins in this way: Either wash the child with a mild *salt solution,* or wrap the child in a towel or shirt *dipped in a solution of salt.* Wrap the child in blankets, put him or her to bed, and cover lightly with bedclothes. The eruptions will soon be visible. Have the child drink lots of water.

This therapy should not be used in lieu of consulting a physician.

Nonbacterial eruptions: Apply shirts or towels that have been dipped in hayflower tea before bedtime every other day for 2 weeks. This will bring out the eruptions and toxins. Have the child drink lots of water.

In both cases, strengthen the child with frequent cold baths or cold spongings, but never allow a child to become chilled!

ADULTS (see also Boils, Eczema, Erysipelas)

Water Therapy

Drink copious amounts of fluids, such as water, fruit juices, vegetable juices (especially carrot juice, parsley, and other alkaline vegetables), peppermint tea, red clover, nettle tea, and burdock tea.

Twice a week for 15 minutes take warm oatstraw baths. Change water twice during the bath. Conclude bath with a 1-minute cold sponging or cold bath.

Three times a week before going to bed, or in the morning upon arising, sponge with cold water for 1 minute.

ERYSIPELAS

Water Therapy

Erysipelas is an acute streptococcal infection of the skin that produces sharp swollen areas. It is often accompanied by fever and general discomfort.

Local discomfort can be relieved by applying cold packs to the area. Throw out the compresses afterward. Also use detoxification therapy.

Acute stage: As soon as you see strange pus postules emerge, and you know you haven't been in touch with poison ivy or poison oak, apply an ice bag continuously over the area. As the disease advances in different areas, apply additional fresh ice bags, since each new area is at an acute stage. Occasionally apply a hot moist compress to the affected area to renew the ability of the tissues to react to the ice bag application.

General Therapy

Erysipelas can cause several severe secondary complications and you may wish to consider using antibiotics. If you do use an antibiotic also eat yogurt or take yogurt or acidopholus tablets to restore the natural intestinal flora of the system.

EYES
(see also Glaucoma, Eye Bath)

A healthy body can throw off unneeded fluids through perspiration and breathing and in the feces and urine. However, in weakened people, fluids that are *not eliminated* sometimes collect in the head. When they do so, the eyes are used as an outlet. Therefore, while eye problems may be treated directly, the whole body must also be treated. If you consistently have eye problems, check for infections in the teeth. Also stimulate the kidney and stomach reflex points.

Water Therapy Techniques for the Eyes

Irrigation: Tepid splashes are excellent for those who read, sew, or do close work, but eye irrigations may be cold, tepid, or hot. Adding milk, comfrey tea, or quince seed to the water often makes long-term irrigation and eye bathing more pleasant. Special eye cups are available in drugstores. You can also use a sterilized whiskey shot glass.

Compresses: These may be hot, cold, or ice, according to the problem. Use thin folds of cotton or a linen handkerchief (not more than 2–3 thicknesses). Thick compresses on the eye become warm too quickly.

Change cold compresses every 5 minutes, especially if there is any inflammation. Hot compresses should be as hot as you can tolerate.

TO IMPROVE VISION

Water Therapy

Splash eyes with cold water each morning for a month.
Apply pot cheese compresses on eye or eyes.
Apply cold horsetail compresses on eye or eyes.

ABRASIONS (or Splits in the Eye)

Water Therapy

After removing caked dirt with a moist gauze, wash out the abrasion with a sterile salt solution (distilled water and sodium chloride). Apply a cold compress immediately.

General Therapy

Heal the abrasion with an opthalmic or calendula ointment.

STY

Water Therapy

A sty is an infection that is usually caused by staphylococci. Bring the sty to a head by applying a hot moist compress of sterile gauze for 10 minutes. Repeat several times a day. Wash hands after each treatment.

General Therapy

Check the teeth for possible infection. Add vitamins A, C, and D to the diet.

PINK EYE (Acute Catarrhal Conjunctivitis)
(watery discharge, itching, burning, smarting of the lids; red lid).

Water Therapy

Pink eye is highly contagious and is usually caused by pneumococci or staphylococci. To strengthen the eye, apply a sterile gauze cold compress for 15 minutes daily. Change the compress every 30 seconds. Antibiotics are often used to control an acute case.

General Therapy

Use only personal towels. Keep the eye free of discharge. Avoid known irritants, carefully remove foreign bodies, and have physician remove any inverted lashes.

FOLICULAR CONJUNCTIVITIS

Water Therapy

Apply a sterile gauze cold compress to the eye several times a day. Change the compress frequently.

FOREIGN BODIES

Water Therapy

Carefully remove the foreign body from the eye. Apply sterile gauze cold compresses, or gently splash the eye with cold water to restore the tone to the tissues. If you have been splashed with lime, acid, or alkalies, splash the eye with cold water and remove any foreign particles. Conclude treatment with hot moist compresses to help with absorption and pain relief.

INFLAMMATION OF THE EYE (Blepharitis)

Water Therapy

Blepharitis is an inflammation of the lid margins that causes redness, thickening, and occasional scales and crusts. It is usually caused by staphylococci.

Hot compresses twice daily help during the acute stage.

Irrigate with cold water, and apply a fresh sterile gauze cold compress every minute for one hour every day during the non-acute stage.

WHITE DISCHARGE IN THE EYE (Children)

Water Therapy

Direct a gentle tepid shower to the head at least once a day. Apply fresh pot cheese poultice to the eye several times a day for 15 minutes at a time.

Several times a day, immerse the child up to his or her armpits in a 2-second cold water bath.

EXERCISE RECOVERY

Water Therapy

Take cayenne pepper (¼ teaspoon in one cup of hot water) *before* stretching to increase circulation, raise body temperature and help muscle flexibility. Very *short* hot application of water, or very brief hot baths are the best means of quickly recovering from exercise exhaustion. Long hot applications or long hot baths will cause muscular weakness. Always end the hot water applications with a toning cold water splash. Each evening before bedtime, tread in cold water for several minutes. This strengthens the body, and prevents postexercise leg cramps.

Hot ginger baths will help to relax stiff muscles. Dissolve small amounts of ginger powder in boiling water and add to the hot bath. Gradually increase the amount of ginger from a teaspoon to a tablespoon, depending on your tolerance.

EXHAUSTION

Water Therapy

Warm baths: When you are feeling even slightly fatigued, take a long warm bath to which aromatic herbs or pine extract have been added. End this bath with an invigorating cold water splash over the entire body. This restores tone to the sedated and relaxed muscles.

Herbs: Add pine extract, aromatic herbs in cheesecloth or a tea infuser to the bathwater, or splash apple cider vinegar over the shoulders, arms, chest, and back. Also place a cup of the vinegar in the bathwater, as it relieves muscle fatigue.

Salt glow: Before getting in the bath, rub the body with a paste of salt and water. Soak in tub. See page 75, Fig. 16.

Brush the feet: While in the bath, brush the feet with a good natural bristle brush or a loofah to stimulate the entire system. There is no organ of the body that cannot be reached through deep foot massage.

Alternate percussion showers: Direct an alternate hot and cold jet shower over the entire body. This acts as a tonic. The hot stream should always last longer than the cold.

Cold baths, cold showers: A brief (3–6 seconds) cold plunge or cold shower spray will energize and tone the entire body. Just treading in cold water, and then kneeling down briefly into the water will revitalize even the most exhausted person.

FATIGUE

GENERAL FATIGUE

Water Therapy

After a long and difficult day, splash apple cider vinegar on your shoulders, neck, and chest. Or add apple cider vinegar to a neutral or warm water bath. While in the bath, wet a wash cloth with the vinegar, apply over chest and back, and then take a relaxing soak in the water up to the chin. During the bath, friction massage the body with a large bath brush, or use a rough wash cloth, loofah, or sponge. Always end the bath with a cold water splash to invigorate the body and a vigorous towel rub.

General Therapy

After rubbing the body dry, lie down on a *slant board* for 10 minutes. This reversal of gravity is very refreshing.

Various drinks are also reviving. Drink grape juice with a dash of cayenne pepper, or peppermint tea with a tiny pinch of ginseng powder. Sometimes a vitamin C or a calcium tablet will restore flagging energy.

FATIGUE IN THE MORNING

Water Therapy

Take frequent 1–2 minute cold half baths (up to the kidney area) to overcome consistent early morning fatigue and "heavy head."

Also, try kneeling and treading in cold water, or splashing cold water on your ankles to give general tone and vigor to your tired system.

Direct a cold jet shower stream to the soles of the feet. As often as possible while in the bath, or after the shower, brush the soles of the feet or knead and tap the soles. This awakens the entire body.

FEET

Water Therapy

See Foot Baths, pages 62–69. Note especially the therapeutic action of hayflower foot baths.

COLD FEET

Water Therapy

Increase the circulation by directing alternate hot and cold showers to the feet. The hot should always last longer than the cold. Repeat each sequence several times each session, up to a dozen times. End with the cold, or apply a jet stream cold shower to the soles of the feet. Dry the feet thoroughly with a rough towel. After several days, even obstinate cases of cold feet respond favorably.

SWOLLEN FEET

Water Therapy

To immediately reduce swelling, wrap the feet in cloths that have been dipped in cold hayflower tea or diluted hayflower extract. Do this once a day. Leave the cloths on for 15 minutes.

Purify the system by sponging the entire body with warm water and apple cider vinegar twice a week. Do not towel dry, but return to bed, lie under the covers, and dry in bed. The water evaporates quickly, and a feeling of pleasant warmth pervades the body.

Every second or third day, early in the morning, apply a cold abdominal compress that has been dipped in apple cider vinegar. You will need a fairly large compress that has been folded 4 times. Wrap a dry cloth over the wet compress, leave compress on and pin dry. Leave compress on until it dries, or overnight. You may walk around with this "girdle." It has a general heating effect.

On alternate days, direct a cold percussion shower to thighs and knees.

PERSPIRATION OF THE FEET

Water Therapy

It is natural and necessary for the body to exude unhealthy substances through the pores of the skin, and especially through the soles of the feet. *Never* close off this avenue of perspiration, as it may cause later illnesses.

If your feet perspire excessively, soak them for several minutes each day in a tepid hayflower bath. Also drink herbal teas to flush the kidneys.

DYE ON FEET

Water Therapy

Walking on wet grass, particularly dewy, wet grass, will cause dyes, paints, etc, to disappear within a few hours.

ACUTE FOOT INFECTION

Immerse infected foot into alternate hot and cold water foot baths. If preferred, apply alternate hot and cold compresses to the foot.

HEEL BRUISE

A heel bruise and the stone bruise of the metatarsal will be extremely tender for many months.

Water Therapy

Add arnica tincture to a neutral foot bath and soak foot for several hours each day. As often as possible, wrap a cold apple cider vinegar compress around the painful area of the foot.

Massage the area with herbal liniments or ointments, such as Olbas, eucalyptus, or wintergreen, that bring the blood to the surface.

SOLE OF THE FOOT INJURY

Common puncture wounds on the sole of the foot must always be checked by a doctor. Do not allow open wounds to become contaminated.

Water Therapy

Soak the foot daily in neutral salt water. Add tincture of St. John's Wort or calendula tincture to water. Ledum tincture is also excellent. The wound should heal in 3–5 days.

FEVER

Chills and fever are not diseases, but a mechanism for raising the body temperature to a new level when the heat balance of the body is disturbed by disease.

Water Therapy

Fever is a natural process. While drugs suppress the fever, water therapy works by lowering the heat, and reducing the production of fever and heat. Effective water therapy includes copious drinking of pure water, internal irrigations with water, an ice cap, external cold sponging, cold friction massages, cold body compresses, cold partial compresses, cold showers and baths, a wet sheet rub, toweling.

Cold Water Drinking

You can reduce temperature due to fever from ½ to 2 degrees by drinking 2–3 pints of cold (40°F or so) water within a 10-minute period. *Drink between 6–7 quarts in 24 hours.*

This simple therapy lowers the body temperature, absorbs the heat, dilutes the blood, causes evaporation on the skin, and activates the kidneys. It also neutralizes and flushes out any poisons in the body, stimulates the liver in its detoxification job and prevents loss of body fluids.

You can also drink sage tea to cleanse the body and help reduce the fever.

Tepid Enemas

Take the enema in the knee-chest position. Use 2–3 pints of tepid water. Retain the water between 5–10 minutes, or *as long as possible.* When the water is expelled it will be warmer, and you will be cooler. Tests by hydrotherapy physicians have proved that this irrigation will lower the temperature half a degree if no other heat production has taken place internally.

Sage tea may be added to the enema water to help lower the fever.

Cold Water Therapies that Combat Fever

Always drink cold water to supplement the following therapies.

1. Damp sheet compress. This is the best of all applications. Use a three-quarter or half compress if you prefer not to have your arms covered. Renew every 5–8 minutes as the sheet will quickly absorb the heat of the body. Packs applied several times a day for short periods are more effective than one pack applied for a long period.

2. Cold friction massage. Spray the body with hot water afterward.

3. Apply a continuous cold abdominal compress. The cold abdominal compress combats fever in this way: When the temperature is high, gastric secretions stop, and the system loses its ability to break down certain materials. The mouth and tongue become hot and dry. The abdominal compress, via reflex action, causes the mouth to become moist and the stomach juices to secrete more normally. This lessens the danger

FEVER CHART

Symptoms	Water Therapy
HIGH TEMPERATURE (normal perspiration)	Wet sheet body compress, cold bath with friction, alternate hot and cold compresses.
PROFUSE PERSPIRATION	Gentle perspiration daub every few minutes. This hastens evaporation, lessens possibility of chill.
NO PERSPIRATION	Sponge bath, or evaporating sheet.
COOL or CLAMMY SKIN	Hot blanket pack or hot moist compress to spine. Follow by cold friction.
BLUE, PALE, COLD SKIN	Use heat and friction to bring blood to surface. Follow by cold rubs to warm up and maintain reaction. Wrap in warm clothing.
GOOSEFLESH	Indicates contraction of the small blood vessels of the skin, preventing heat elimination. Apply hot compresses to spine. Follow with cool water friction on spine and rest of the body.
CARDIAC WEAKNESS	Cold compress over the heart. Cold sponging of the spine and general body. Cold friction massage. Care must be exerted with heart patients to prevent a sudden rush of blood to the heart. This is achieved with general cold friction, and repeated cold compresses.
HEATSTROKE	Wet sheet, cold bath. Simultaneous massage. See p. 208.
SUNSTROKE	Ice therapy and massage. Cold compresses to heart, forehead, and head. See p. 208.
INTESTINAL PERFORATION 1. Infants	Tepid baths, cooling packs, cool friction massage. Do *not* use cold.
2. Elderly	Avoid shock. Use prolonged tepid bath, wet sheet rubbing, pack in wet sheet.
TYPHOID FEVER, TYPHUS	Few seconds in cold bath with friction rubbing. This is the Brand Bath technique.
ERUPTIONS (measles, scarlet fever)	Treat in same way as all fevers, but eruption period can be limited by utilizing neutral alkaline baths, such as oatmeal or bicarbonate of soda, every 15 minutes. Salt wash or wraps.
URINE SUPPRESSION (during eruptive fever)	Drink great amounts of water. Enema at 80°F-90°F 2 times a day. Blanket pack for 20–30 minutes. Follow with cold compress, covered with dry cloth, on thighs.

of any complication occurring from the fever. Change the compress as often as it becomes hot, every 30 minutes or so.

4. Apply alternate hot and cool compresses. This will reduce body heat, lessen fever, stimulate the surface of the skin, and aid elimination.

5. Daub continuously with cold wet cloths to absorb perspiration.

6. Use cold sprays.

7. Apply a cold compress to the spine, head and neck, or abdomen.

8. Take a tepid enema.

9. Cold sponge bath with water or diluted apple cider vinegar.

10. Cold air bath.

11. Prolonged tepid bath. End with a cool splash.

12. Wash body with cool sage tea. Sage tea is an antiseptic and may also be used to wash the sickroom and the bed.

FINGER PROBLEMS

CRUSHED FINGER

Water Therapy

Place the injured finger in cold water, and keep in the water until the pain disappears. Add fresh cold water or ice water from time to time to keep the water cold. If preferred, a continuous cold compress may be applied.

SPORTS INJURIES

There are many ways to injure fingers during sports activities. Among the injuries are blisters, knuckle scrapes, knuckles bit or injured by human teeth, cuts, nail injuries, sprains, dislocations, and fractures.

Water Therapy

Apply an ice compress or miniature icebag immediately to control bleeding and prevent swelling. Treat with ice for 30 minutes at a time. Apply over finger splint.

Soak any open finger wounds in rosemary tea right away. This promotes healing.

In between ice applications, apply arnica lotion or diluted arnica tincture to unbroken skin wounds. This reduces the pain. Olbas herbal oil or lotion also promotes healing.

Immerse finger or arm in neutral bath. These partial baths quicken healing.

See Resource List for useful aids.

FINGER ABSCESS (Felon)

Water Therapy

Treat this infection in the same way you treat a boil.

To reduce inflammation once the felon has started, immerse entire hand and arm in a hot hand bath of 105°F–130°F for 15 minutes. Repeat several times a day.

FINGER CUT BY PAPER

Water Therapy

Wet finger and place cut area into powdered cloves. This immediately reduces the pain.

FIRST AID
(see Bruises, Hemorrhages, and Wounds and listings for specific body injuries.)

FLU

Flu sufferers who drink copious quantities of herbal teas and pure water, and who use perspiration-inducing detoxification procedures, rarely have complications resulting from the flu.

Water Therapy

Cold compresses, including the damp sheet compress with garlic "paint" on the soles of the feet, hot detoxification baths, drinking of herbal teas, and kidney flushing are all effective water remedies for the flu.

Kidney Flushing

Drink sage tea, with Indian corn silk and a pinch of rue. Use 3 parts sage, 2 parts corn silk, 1 part rue. The sage and the corn silk strengthen the kidneys, and help them to expel large quantities of fluid from the system. Rue speeds up the blood circulation.

Herbal Flu Preventers

Ginseng is an energizer and rebalancer, and helps offset the flu. Add it to hot herbal drinks, or swallow a capsule of the pure powder.

Drink peppermint tea laced with smaller amounts of elderflower and yarrow. Used together they promote perspiration.

Cayenne pepper rebalances the body. You can effectively abort the flu by adding cayenne pepper to any hot herbal drink.

Take a tablespoon of common salt, or sea salt, and a tablespoon of cayenne pepper powder. Mix together. Add a cup of boiling water. When the mixture cools, add a half cup of apple cider vinegar. Drink in ¼ teaspoon doses every few hours before and during flu epidemics. If you have a sensitive stomach, make chamomile tea and use chamomile tea instead of the water. This is strong stuff, but it works fantastically!

Apply a damp sheet compress—either full or three-quarter. Before turning the ends of the sheet up around the feet, coat the feet with vaseline (it has the right viscosity), and "paint" the *soles* of the feet (no other part!) with blended or mashed garlic that has been blended into vaseline. *Cover the feet with the sheet and the blanket.* The garlic paint can sometimes turn the tide in a serious illness.

Baths

Take any of the hot detoxification baths. Apple cider vinegar baths (hot or neutral water) will relieve body soreness. Half or full hot baths relieve body aches, and inspire perspiration. Apply a cold compress to the head, and drink either hot lemonade or hot pineapple juice during the bath.

Between baths, stimulate the heart by applying a cold compress to heart area.

Pneumonia

Apply a cold compress to the chest between the hot baths, and wear a cold abdominal compress continuously between treatments. Change this compress every 20 minutes or whenever it becomes warm. Used together, these applications overcome head congestion and stimulate the diaphragm.

Flu and Fever

In addition to the details outlined under "Fever," pages 152–154, flu sufferers should:

Perspire freely, but do not become chilled.

Take an enema as soon as possible.

Divert blood flow away from the head and chest with either a hot full bath (use a cold compress on forehead) or a hot leg bath with simultaneous hot moist compresses on throat or chest or spine (use a cold compress on forehead).

Drink hot lemonade or hot pineapple juice.

As soon as the perspiration starts, take a tepid shower, and gradually make the water hotter and hotter, according to your body's tolerance. Use a cold compress on the forehead during the shower. Constantly renew this compress, as otherwise the shower can weaken the body.

The following morning, relieve the aching of the back and limbs with a simultaneous hot leg pack and hot moist compress applied to the spine. Conclude the treatment with a vigorous cold friction massage.

After these treatments, only treat with *tonic* measures such as the cold friction massage, or cold towel rub, or an alternate hot and cold spray shower directed to the spine and legs (always conclude with cold shower).

General Therapy

After the flu, build up your body with alfafa sprouts, sesame seeds, fresh herbs, fresh fruits and vegetables—especially beets—and grape juice. Add liberal pinches of cayenne pepper to drinks and food.

FOOT
(see Feet)

FRACTURES

Fractures must be set by a professional.

Water Therapy

While waiting for the physician to arrive, or on the way to the hospital, fractures may be contained by applying ice bags. This controls internal bleeding.

Later during rehabilitation, you can improve blood circulation in arm and wrist fractures by frequently immersing the entire arm in hot water for 3 minutes, and then in cold water for 30 seconds. Repeat 3 times. Continue therapy as long as needed to restore normal mobility.

FROSTBITE

Frostbite is the destruction of the skin by freezing.

Water Therapy

Rush victim to hospital. If this is not possible, rewarm a frostbitten limb in high temperature water. The U.S. Navy says water of 102°F–105°F will bring excellent results. Because there may be tissue damage if the thawing is too slow or too fast, *use a thermometer to monitor the process.* If you haven't a thermometer, see page 103.

Another technique is to keep the frostbitten limb covered with a wool or flannel blanket, and warm all other parts of the body. Create maximum circulation by rubbing the limb vigorously.

In 30 minutes, a flush usually returns to the skin. The thawed tissues can then be soaked in a whirlpool bath for 20 minutes once or twice a day until the healing is complete.

Children: Wrap a compress that has been soaked in neutral water and strained hayflower tea over the affected part. Cover the wet compress with a dry cloth.

Take a series of hand or foot baths with one-quarter vinegar and three-quarters cold water.

General Therapy

During very cold weather, always wear a hat. An uncovered head quickly gives away body heat. Wear mittens instead of gloves. Wear long johns, wool sweaters, and other warm clothing. Wet clothing, fatigue, and a couple of drinks too many can make you more susceptible to frostbite.

GENITAL INFLAMMATION

Water Therapy

Apply and renew a cold genital compress (see page 41) every 15 minutes.

GENITAL PROBLEMS
(sports injuries)

BLOWS TO THE TESTICLES

Water Therapy

Blows to this area are indicated by a sudden ashen pallor, acute pain, and nausea.

Immediately apply ice packs. If bleeding continues, put athlete to bed, give additional support to the testes, and apply ice packs intermittently. Sponge area with strong rosemary tea. When pain subsides, apply a hot compress. Alternate the hot compress with short cold spongings.

General Therapy

The testes should be examined by a physician within minutes of the injury if symptoms do not subside immediately. Even if they do subside, a physician or urologist should be consulted. The area may take months to reabsorb blood. After such an injury it is important to add additional cup support.

Fitted supporters are now mandatory in professional and intercollegiate sports, but not for very young players. Physicians dealing with sports injuries strongly advise the use of such supporters for all ages.

ROTATED TESTES

Water Therapy

After treatment by a urologist, cold sit baths and a genital compress will strengthen the area.

General Therapy

This rotation is rather rare, but it can occur in contact sports, particularly to men in their teens and twenties. The testes can sometimes be rotated into a 180° turn. Consult a urologist for any such testicular pain and swelling or rotation.

GLANDS

SWEAT GLANDS

Water Therapy

The skin is the largest, as well as one of the most complex, organs in the body. It acts through sweat glands to eliminate normal fluids, and to regulate the heat of the body through perspiration.

As a preventive measure before or during illness, the skin *can be forced* to take over the function of other organs, such as the liver. This is accomplished by *stimulating perspiration* through detoxifying baths such as hayflower, sage, or nutmeg. Nutmeg, in particular, can stimulate inactive sweat glands. Various body compresses, particularly the damp sheet compress, can also stimulate sweat glands.

SALIVARY GLANDS

Water Therapy

Apply cold compresses to malfunctioning glands to increase their function and restore normal activity.

LYMPH GLANDS

Water Therapy

Inactive lymph circulation responds to cold water application and massage. The best massage is a professional Swedish massage, as this increases normal circulation in the area.

Swollen glands on the neck respond to a cold double compress. Dip the compress into cold rosemary tea and apply. The rosemary alleviates pain and reduces the pressure of the swollen glands. Apply a second, larger, dry wool or flannel compress on top.

GLAUCOMA
(see also Eyes)

Water Therapy

Localized disturbances in the eyes can be somewhat helped by water treatments that may also help to reduce the vascular tension.

Simultaneously apply ice bags over the carotid arteries and take either a hot foot bath or a hot leg bath.

Keeping ice bags on, end the treatment with a cold friction massage of the legs or an alternate hot and cold percussion shower directed to the feet.

Keep the bowels open with a laxative diet, abdominal massage, and water irrigation.

However, water therapy does not replace proper medical supervision and treatment of the eyes.

GOITER

Water Therapy

Several times a day, simultaneously apply an ice bag on the heart area and another ice bag on goiter area. Leave ice bags on for 30–60 minutes.

Use a cold friction massage 1–3 times a day on the entire body. This restores normal body tone and checks overactivity of the sweat glands.

If the feet are consistently cold, apply frequent alternate hot and cold showers to the feet, or take alternate hot and cold foot baths. The hot application should be longer than the cold, but always end with the cold.

GROIN STRAIN
(sports injuries)

Water Therapy

In sports, the complaint of a "tight" groin is so common that it is often ignored, and frequently leads to a disability that is even more difficult to cure, and can last several weeks. This, in turn, may cause a season-long problem, or one that persists throughout all future athletic activity.

Immediately apply an ice bag to the area, and hold in place with an elastic bandage wound in a figure 8.

After the bleeding stops, use a program of alternate long hot and short cold showers to increase circulation to the area. Direct shower to area of pain. Occasional or nightly application of a double cold abdominal compress will reinvigorate and tone the area, and have a general heating effect.

General Therapy

After the initial water therapy, the athlete must suspend play until the bleeding stops. During the healing process, use ointments and liniments that bring blood to the surface. These include wintergreen liniment, Olbas lotion or ointment, arnica lotion, mustard plaster, cayenne pepper or ginger powder poultice.

Dr. Vincent Di Stephano, team physician for the Philadelphia Eagles, says he uses hot moist compresses as a secondary treatment if stiffness persists in the groin area.

Sitting in a cold whirlpool sit bath also helps.

An excellent preventive exercise that is used especially by skiers is to lift one foot to a table, or bathroom sink, and stretch the groin area by leaning forward a half dozen times.

HAND INJURIES
(see also Arm Injuries)

Water Therapy

Plunge the hand into containers of alternate hot and cold water. Plunge into hot water for 2–3 minutes and into cold water for 30 seconds. Repeat 6 times.

Neutral partial baths of the hand or arm will encourage the healing of any finger, hand, or arm injury.

HARDENING OF THE ARTERIES
(see Arteries)

HAY FEVER

Water Therapy

Drink copious amounts of fluid, especially apple cider vinegar and honey mixed with water. Mix 1 tablespoon of each into a cup of water.

Tone digestive organs with frequent daytime applications of the cold abdomen compress. Renew compress every 3 hours.

Occasionally during the week, use these foot applications: hot leg baths and alternate hot and cold footbaths. Use the wet stocking therapy during sleep hours.

HEADACHES

Headaches can be symptoms of an internal body problem, or they can be caused by controllable outside forces. It is not only useful but imperative to check, and when possible, eliminate the *causal* agents. Headaches that are generated from within the body may be due to digestive problems such as sluggish liver, indigestion, constipation, inflammation of the stomach; kidney or bowel problems; high blood pressure; or anemia. Outside factors include such diverse causes as sun glare, overheated or underventilated rooms, or tiny gas leaks from a heater, stove, or dryer.

HEADACHES

There are three types of headaches: functional, organic, and circulatory.

Causes	Therapy

Functional Headaches

ACUTE TOXIC HEADACHE
Drug poisoning
Infection
Acute nephritis
Uremia

Institute immediate and vigorous treatment of causative factors.

Relieve congestion with ice bags to carotid arteries and base of head.

CHRONIC TOXIC HEADACHE
Rheumatism
Arthritis
Gout
Sluggish liver

Finding the causative factor is important. Water measures should be *tonic and eliminative,* but may take weeks or months to overcome the problem, since it is chronic.

Wrap calf of the leg from ankle to knee in single folded cloth dipped in fuller's earth and water. It can remain on for several hours. Blood is taken from the head and ache disappears.

Alternate hot and cold compresses to head are generally soothing. Single cold compresses will also be helpful.

Go outdoors, walk, sit in sunshine during early morning or late afternoon, but always be careful of overexposure.

Investigate pressure therapy, manipulative therapy. Massage head frequently.

MIGRAINE

This problem only responds to long range *tonic* and *eliminative* water therapy. Check into reflex points of liver, stomach, and pelvis, and concentrate shower stream on these points.

Working outdoors may be helpful.

Organic Headaches

MENINGITIS

Water therapy is not totally satisfactory here because of the intracranial pressure.

Use methods to *divert* the head congestion.

Circulatory Headaches

ANEMIA

Alternate hot and cold compresses to head. Repeat daily, or on alternate days.

Apply cold friction massage to body.

Both of these stimulate circulation.

Table continued on page 162

HEADACHES

Causes	Therapy
TOO MUCH CONGESTION (hyperemic)	Deplete blood supply with either: 1. Fan shower to feet for 1 minute. Massage neck and shoulders and rest. 2. Hot foot baths, ice bags to carotid arteries (large arteries of neck). Either of these tend to give relief.
CONGESTION DUE TO TOXEMIA or CONGESTION FROM STUDYING TOO HARD, OR CONCENTRATING TOO HARD	Use either alternate hot and cold leg bath or alternate hot and cold percussion shower to feet.
PASSIVE CONGESTION (as from a cold)	Same as for anemia—alternate hot and cold compress to head. Follow with hot foot bath or hot leg pack. Finish with cold friction massage or cold percussion shower to feet. The brain is very sensitive to overcongestion. Therefore, applications to the feet ending with *cold* overcome the passive congestion, and keep the blood flow away from the head.

HEAD CONGESTION

Water Therapy

When I am working hard on any project that requires sustained energy and clear thinking, I frequently walk in a half bath of cold water for a few minutes, or sit in the cold bath water for a few seconds. Both these techniques relieve brain fatigue.

Reflex Points for Head

Use short cold water applications to hands, head, or feet. Short cold showers or brief cold shallow sit baths are also helpful.

HEART PROBLEMS

The objective of water therapy in acute heart problems is to sustain vital activity and to stimulate the heart by either reflex or direct action. Many physicians feel that some heart problems are due to reflex action from the stomach, and urge that this area receive exceptional attention.

Always consult a physician for any heart troubles. You may use water therapy as secondary therapy for heart problems.

Water Therapy

The ice bag is one of the most efficient tonics for the heart. Cold friction massage treatment, however, has the greatest *range* of use in treating organic heart problems. It can be used from the initial acute stage all through the recovery period. A prolonged, fan, no-pressure, neutral shower over the heart *slows* the heart beat and *strengthens* the organ. Slapping the chest with a cold towel *increases* heart rate and force.

Note: When ice is placed over the heart, indications of collapse rapidly disappear.

General Therapy

Massage the pinky of the left hand, and massage the area directly over the pinky up the entire arm, and across the breast to about the level of the nipple. This is the acupuncture heart meridian.

Also massage the fleshy parts of each thumb.

ACUTE SHOCK

In the event no physician is available, the following techniques may be used, along with artificial respiration, to treat shock. These water therapies involve a change of temperature to increase stimulation.

Water Therapy

Place a hot moist compress on the heart area for 2 minutes. Dry gently. Massage the area with ice for 30 seconds. Dry gently. Repeat this sequence 3–4 times. After the 4th time, rub the area vigorously with the hand. Apply a cold compress that has been dipped in full-strength or diluted apple cider vinegar.

If ice cubes aren't available, slap the chest with a cold wet towel along with each inhalation movement of artificial respiration. See chart page 197.

MYOCARDITIS

Myocarditis is an inflammation of the muscle of the heart.

Water Therapy

Cold has an inhibitory effect on the motor stimulating nerves, and an ice pack, placed over the heart for 36–72 hours, will give the inflamed and strained heart the best opportunity to recover.

ACUTE ENDOCARDITIS

Acute endocarditis is associated with rheumatic fever.

Water Therapy

Renew cold compresses on the heart every 15 minutes.

Apply sectional sponging of the body with cold water and *moderate* friction 3 times a day.

After inflammation is reduced: Use passive exercise, or sectional cold friction massage.

Apply an ice bag to the heart for 30 minutes 4–5 times a day.

Lightly massage the body.

Before lunch: Use any tonic treatment such as cold friction massage, cold towel rub, hot foot bath, hot moist compresses to the spine, or alternate hot and cold showers or jet streams directed to spine.

Two hours after lunch or two hours after supper: Release tensions built up during the day with an alternate hot and cold foot bath. Always end with cold.

When pulse is normal: Rest much of the time, but begin regular walking exercises. Use only 3 stimulating water treatments a week. The evening treatment should be sedative. Tonic treatments that are useful include an occasional salt massage before a bath, and an alternate hot and cold shower on feet and legs.

UNUSUAL HEART RHYTHM (Tachycardia)

Tachycardia is a slow or fast heart beat.

Make sure to clear up any digestive problems, especially constipation or indigestion.

Water Therapy

Use the cold mitten friction massage in 15-minute treatments. At the same time, apply an ice bag over the heart area and at the nape of the neck. Repeat treatment hourly if needed.

ANGINA

Water Therapy

Water therapy is to be used in addition to all other medical treatments.

Apply a hot moist compress over the heart area for one minute. Immediately follow with a cold compress. Leave the cold compress on for five minutes.

Apply the alternate hot and cold compresses for several hours if necessary, as this can frequently ease an acute attack.

Instant pain relief: 15-second hot hand baths or hot foot baths relieve the pain. The water can be very hot—to tolerance or 120°F. Repeat every 5 minutes until there is an improvement.

EDEMA (Swollen tissues)

Water Therapy

Plunge legs into alternate hot and cold foot baths that contain enough water to cover any swollen area. Alternate the baths 10 times. The hot water plunge should last 1–2 minutes; the cold water plunge 10–15 seconds. In the early part of the treatment, the cold water can range from 50°F–70°F. Later on, add chunks of ice to the water. Dry after each cold treatment.

If only the *ankle* is swollen, you can either massage or use a vibrator on the area.

HEARTBURN

Permanent relief from heartburn can be achieved by increasing the tone in the stomach, intestines, and the whole system.

Water Therapy

Every day, sponge the abdomen with diluted apple cider vinegar, *or,* several times a week, apply neutral hayflower or diluted apple cider vinegar compresses on the abdomen for 1½ hours.

Each week take several very brief cold half baths.

For relief of heartburn, prepare a weak wormwood tea and drink a spoonful every hour.

Children: Chamomile tea is a pleasant and mild digestive aid.

Place child in a warm hayflower bath for 9–10 minutes. Conclude bath with a cold sponging and a friction drying.

An alternative treatment is to apply a towel that has been dipped in hot hayflower tea. Wrap the towel around the child from the armpits to the knees. Cover the child with a light blanket for 1½ hours.

HEEL
(see Feet)

HEMORRHAGE
(while waiting for a doctor to arrive)

MILD BLEEDING

Water Therapy

At no time should heat in any form be applied to any acute injury. Mild bleeding, except on the feet and hands, responds to alternate hot and cold *hand* baths. In general, applying ice plus *pressure* on the wound with a sterile cloth, or finger pressure on the nearest artery, will stop the bleeding and the subsequent build-up of fluid in the tissues.

Herb Aids

In addition to ice and compression therapy, there are several herbs that can be used for excessive bleeding:

A diluted tincture of calendula (pot marigold) petals, or the juice of the petals *(Succus Calendula)* has an antiseptic and healing effect on wounds. The ointment is also effective in healing scars and bruises.

Cayenne pepper smarts on a wound, but it is *extremely* effective. Use cayenne in powder form on wounds or add a small amount to ½ cup of hot water and drink.

MILD BODY BLEEDING (in areas other than hands or feet)

Alternate hot and cold hand baths.

BLEEDING IN ABDOMEN, INTESTINES, STOMACH, PELVIC AREA

Apply a single cold compress on *trunk.* Replace the compress as soon as it becomes warm. An ice bag placed on the area over a local hemorrhage intensifies compress action. Swallow cracked ice. A small amount of cayenne pepper powder in ½ cup of hot water will often control internal bleeding. *Get to a hospital as soon as possible.*

ARTERY BLEEDING

In addition to local pressure, steam-laden air sometimes acts as a styptic.

General Therapy

Firm pressure is the best method of controlling most bleeding wounds. Apply pressure on wound with a sterile bandage, or apply firm pressure to the artery. Hold 10 minutes and release slowly. Go to the hospital.

CEREBRAL BLEEDING

If no physician is available, use this early treatment: Gently place an ice bag or a helmet of ice on the head. Also apply ice bags or ice compresses to *back of the neck,* and over the *carotid artery* (large artery on neck that ends near ear.)

Keep limbs warm with hot water bottle.

Keep applications in place until hemorrhage is over. Absolute rest and keeping perfectly still are essential.

LABOR

When Bleeding Is Slight After Delivery

Use a hot vaginal douche (alum powder or witch hazel may be added to the water).

Use ice bag continuously on the pubic area.

Drink red raspberry leaf tea, before, during, and after labor.

HEMORRHOIDS

Most hemorrhoids are not merely local problems, but are usually an indication of a body disturbance, possibly in the liver, and the blood brought to the liver.

Water Therapy

Pain: Use heat to relieve spasm. The hot shallow sit bath is the most effective of all available hot applications. If facilities are not available for such baths, apply hot moist compresses to the area.

Hot foot baths or bidet-type upward showers are also helpful.

Bleeding: Use ice as a styptic, and apply cold compresses on the vertebrae between the hips and on the perineum (the area between the anus and scrotum or vagina). This checks the blood flow.

Long range: Wear a T-shaped cold genital compress to bed, and occasionally use all of these cold therapies: prolonged cold shallow sit bath, ice bag to the perineum, and alternate hot and cold perineal shower spray.

Drink plenty of water, herb teas, and juice.

General Therapy

Take vitamin C and vitamin E. Avoid refined foods and sugars. Walk, stretch, and get plenty of exercise—especially if you have a sedentary job.

HERNIA (CHILDREN)

Water Therapy

Kneipp used the following water therapies for children's hernia:

Wrap the child in a towel dipped in fresh pine extract and neutral to cold water. Cover the area from the armpits to the knees. Apply for 1½ hours.

Alternate treatment with 1 hour applications of a neutral compress that has been dipped in hayflower tea to the stomach area.

Once a day wash the child in cold water.

To strengthen the child, each day for a week direct a mild stream of water to different areas of the body. Concentrate on only *one area at a time.* Start with showers to the upper part of the back, then sponge the entire body. Toward the end of the week *sit* the child in several inches of cold water for a few seconds. After this, start the child walking in cold water as often as possible. Occasionally direct a mild stream of water to the knee area.

Check with your physician or pediatrician. This water therapy treatment does *not* replace such medical attention and supervision.

HIVES

Hives are local eruptions caused by drug allergy, insect stings or bites, or the eating of certain foods, particularly shellfish, eggs, nuts, and fruits. The hives may follow severe viral or streptococcal infections, or be a result of a chronic infection (check dental abscesses for instance).

Water Therapy

Hives may be somewhat relieved by drinking large amounts of water, and irrigating the body with an enema to help get rid of waste materials.

A dry hot pack, which can be used even for the very young, will create heavy perspiration, drain off the irritating substances, and also stimulate the liver and the kidneys.

HYDROCHLORIC ACID
(deficiency)

Hydrochloric acid(HCl) is an essential acid in the digestive process. Researchers have discovered that frequently, after about 25 years, the body produces less of this acid. Some persons 50 years of age or more may have a greatly depleted supply of hydrochloric acid, as their systems have slowed down even more.

Some cancer therapy specialists feel that the body's production of this substance must be supplemented, and advise taking HCl tablets after each meal. HCl tablets buffered with the enzymes betaine or pepsin are available in most health food stores.

Anyone with a peptic or stomach ulcer should not take HCL tablets.

Water Therapy

Improve the general tone in the abdominal area. A short time before meals, apply a cold compress on the upper middle stomach area for 10 minutes. Each night, apply a double cold abdominal compress (this has a heating effect).

Continue these treatments, and drink 2 glasses of cold water 1 hour before breakfast until constipation, flatulence, burping, or indigestion symptoms are eliminated.

INDIGESTION

ACUTE INDIGESTION

Check with a physician to make sure the indigestion attack is not related to a problem with your heart.

Water Therapy

Immediate relief: Drink copious quantities of *warm* water. This acts as an emetic. Afterward, drink additional warm water to cleanse the stomach and dilute the acids of decomposition. To quiet the stomach, drink either peppermint, chamomile, or linden tea. Take an enema with chamomile tea or pure, undiluted, noninstant coffee. The coffee enema detoxifies and cleanses the colon.

If pain is severe: Apply hot moist compresses over the area of pain. Renew every 10 minutes.

If vomiting: While it is a great relief to discharge the food that is causing the distress, sometimes vomiting has to be controlled. If this is the case, apply an ice bag over the upper middle region of the stomach, and dry heat such as a hot water bottle on the vertebrae between the shoulders.

Prevention: Drink chamomile tea or peppermint tea. For trips carry either spirit of peppermint or pure peppermint oil. Add a dozen drops of peppermint spirit or oil to hot water to relieve spasms.

Wear a cold double abdominal compress. This is both a specific for acute attacks and a long-range strengthener for digestive organs. It has a general heating effect.

General Therapy

If you sense that you are going to have trouble with digestion, fast for a day or two on nonsprayed apples, apple juice, or on pure bottled water.

CHRONIC INDIGESTION

Water therapy is an adjunct to good diet, careful chewing of foods, and exercise. The proper sequence of water therapy can greatly increase the tone of the body and the capacity of the body to digest and absorb nutrients.

Water Therapy

In general, take frequent showers, starting with a few seconds of a gentle neutral stream and concluding with a few seconds of a neutral jet stream. Direct the showers to the *upper middle stomach* and to the area slightly below.

On arising: *One hour before* the morning meal, sip a glass of *lukewarm* water. Or, if you produce an *excess of hydrochloric acid,* drink hot water on arising. Flex knees and vigorously massage abdomen for 5 minutes, or until gurgling is heard and the water passes from the stomach into the intestines.

After drinking the water, take a 10-minute neutral bath (95°F–98°F.) Conclude bath with tonic friction sponging, sectional cold mitten rub, or cold shower.

In the evening: Several hours after the evening meal, and before going to bed, apply a cold double abdominal compress. In the morning, wash the abdomen with cold water. The compress relieves congested conditions throughout the alimentary canal by drawing blood to the surface.

INFECTION
(see individual listings)

INFLAMMATION
MINOR INFLAMMATION

Water Therapy
Early stage: Prolonged cold water applications are effective in treating minor inflammation. Apply an ice bag over the inflammation, or immerse the inflamed part in extremely cold water or ice water.

Make a paste of fuller's earth (obtained in drugstores). Spread thickly on cloth and bind on the area of inflammation. Renew as soon as dry or heat increases.

Later stage: Apply hot moist compresses, immerse inflamed part in hot bath, or use neutral jet shower or neutral dousing.

If no throbbing pain: Immerse inflamed area in alternate hot and cold partial baths.

INTERNAL DEEP INFLAMMATION

Water Therapy
Note: In treating pleurisy pain, only use *heat.* In treating mastoiditis, heat *must* be used because even the slightest cold application increases the pain.

In soft tissues: Use cold applications

Bony sections: Use hot applications (as in mastoid bone behind the ear)

Abscess: Apply a hot moist compress over the inflammation. Heat alone relieves the pain, but the action doesn't last very long. Therefore, also apply ice bag over large artery supplying blood to the painful area.

Anus, scrotum, prostate, hemorrhoid: Renew cold compress every 15 minutes. At night use T-shaped genital or hemorrhoid compress.

INFLAMMATION CHART

Inflammation or Congestion in This Area	Apply Water here
EYE	Apply hot or cold to side of face, or forehead. This dilates some of the terminal superficial branches of the carotids and depletes the deeper branches.
PHARYNX AND LARYNX	Apply a cold double compress to neck. This depletes the deeper organs and congests the surface vessels.
LUNGS	Apply either to feet and lower limbs, skin surface of the trunk of the body, hips, hands, arms, or shoulders.
PLEURISY	Where congestion is limited, as in pleurisy, hot moist compress can be used directly, as this dilates the posterior, lateral and anterior cutaneous branches of the intercostal arteries, thereby withdrawing blood from the inflamed pleura.
ACUTE CONGESTION	Hot leg double stimulating compress, or full hot blanket, and cold compress, or ice to lobe affected.
KIDNEY	Circulation in these organs decreased by *hot* application to the *back,* as this dilates the posterior branches of the lumbar and lower intercostal arteries. 1. Use hot moist compresses over the lower dorsal and lumbar spine for *entire width of back.* 2. Or use above with ice bag lower third of breast bone (sternum).
STOMACH	Large applications centering at the middle lower abdomen, and extending over the lower chest and sides of the abdomen.
PELVIC ORGANS (bladder, uterus, ovaries, tubes, rectum and prostate)	*Acute:* Start with hot vaginal douche. Use simultaneous water therapy: ice bag to groin, and hot leg, or hot leg and hip pack. Continue 20–30 minutes. Follow with cold mitten friction to the area. Repeat 2–3 times a day, if necessary. *Chronic:* Use hot sit bath, gradually lowering the temperature until it is quite cold, stay in bath a few seconds to minutes. Use alternate hot and cold vaginal douche irrigation frequently. Also use tonic friction methods, and alternate hot and cold showers to lower back, legs and feet.
SPINE (simple congestion)	Hot moist compresses to the spine. This diverts the blood to the arteries supplying the skin and muscles of the back from spinal arteries.
BRAIN	1. Hot leg bath, with cold compress to head. 2. Hot moist compress to face, ears, forehead (except nose). Simultaneously apply ice bags to two carotid arteries, base of brain, top of head. 3. Compress to head, and ice bags to carotid arteries.
MIDDLE EAR and MASTOID	Apply very hot leg bath, hot moist cloths to mastoid bone, simultaneous ice bag over carotid artery, same side as pain for 20–30 minutes. Follow with vigorous cold mitten friction massage to trunk and limbs.
MASTOIDITIS (inflammation of the mastoid bone)	Heat *decreases* pain of inflammation of bony areas. (Ice on the mastoid will increase pain.)

Eye: Use a cold compress.

Face: Spray with cold water or apply cold compresses.

Children: Dip the child in cold water up to his armpits several times a day, and apply a cold water compress that has been folded into thirds or a single cold water and apple cider vinegar compress to inflammation every half hour.

To reduce internal heat, each day give the child a teaspoon of cold-pressed vegetable oil. Also give a spoonful of cold water every half hour.

For finger inflammation, *treat the entire body.* Once a day apply a shirt that has been dipped in tepid hayflower tea and sponge the child's entire body with cold water. Also immerse the child in cold half baths whenever convenient.

INSOMNIA
(see also Sleep)

Water Therapy

Neutral and warm tub baths calm and sedate the body.

A hot moist compress applied to the head for a few minutes produces *drowsiness.*

Alternate hot and cold leg baths will reduce congestion in the head, and help with sleep problems.

When you are awakened in the middle of the night and cannot go back to sleep, run 6–8 inches of cold water in the bathtub. Sit in the shallow cold bath for a minute or two, preferably with your feet on a rubber pillow. Do not dry your body, but go back to bed under covers. This cold bath may be used two or three times a week.

There are many herbal teas that will help quiet the body. Chamomile, linden and sage are all excellent nighttime drinks. You may add honey in small quantities. Hot milk and honey is another old folk remedy that is remarkably effective in calming the body.

Long Range Help

Follow tonic and body strengthening instructions. Cold water plunges, full sponging in cold water, and cold water treading will all prove very helpful in conquering insomnia.

ITCHING, SMARTING, BURNING, PRICKLING
(see also Eczema, Hives, Jockstrap Itch, and Vaginitis)

Water Therapy

Itching caused by hives or heat rashes, numbness and tingling, burning and smarting, or the feeling of insects crawling, can be contained and controlled by the following:

Immersion of entire body or itching part in either cold water or ice water

Application of an ice bag on the area of itching

Very hot sponging
Medicated compresses (vinegar, witch hazel)
Pastes of oatmeal, fenugreek, comfrey, or bicarbonate of soda
Vinegar baths or vinegar sponging
Witch hazel sponging
Neutral salt baths
Bicarbonate of soda baths
Alcohol rub
Short sweating baths, followed by a neutral soap sponging and cool bath

INVALIDS

Water Therapy

Use tonic and tonic friction methods, and also once a week *only* apply a shirt dipped in either hayflower water or fuller's earth and water. Wear it to bed, and cover it with a blanket. This is a strong action but a very successful one.

Frequently splash body with apple cider vinegar.

JET LAG

Water Therapy

On long trips it's very important to drink 1 glass of water for every hour you are in the air. This prevents dehydration, and helps overcome the trauma of jet lag.

Before the plane lands, splash your face with cold water, and brush your teeth. This energizes and revives the entire system. If you are tired, fill the sink with cold water, and plunge your hands in cold water for one minute. Dry vigorously.

General Therapy

During the flight avoid alcohol, and eat lightly—especially on very long trips. Too much food and alcohol impedes sleep. On long trips take along an inflatable neck pillow.

JOCKSTRAP ITCH

Flareups of this ringworm infection occur more often in the summer, and may be brought on by tight clothing. This itch is sometimes complicated by secondary infections and methods of treatment.

Water Therapy

Observe the highest standards of personal cleanliness, as this fungus may persist *indefinitely* on the skin, or may repeatedly infect susceptible individuals.

For acute flareups, apply potassium permanganate compresses.

Use plenty of soap and water, germicide, and ointment, and when bathing be sure to rinse away all soap, and to carefully dry the area. Wear cotton underwear. Boil it after each wearing.

KIDNEY PROBLEMS

ACUTE NEPHRITIS

Water Therapy

Drink large quantities of pure water, high alkaline soups, cranberry juice, watermelon juice, and raw vegetable juices.

Apply a cold compress to the head, immerse the body in a hot half bath, and drink hot lemonade while in the bath. Follow the bath with a 1-quart hot enema, and repeat the enema every 2 hours after the bath until the kidney is flushed and there is a flow of urine. This therapy works when even the strongest drugs fail.

If the kidneys still need stimulation, use the hot pack or hot blanket pack. However, since these tend to be weakening therapies, apply only for a half hour, and watch the pulse and heart action. To protect the heart, apply a large ice bag over the heart area during the pack treatment.

General Therapy

Add large supplements of vitamin A (50,000–75,000 I.U.) and vitamin E (up to 1,000 I.U., providing there is no heart disease or high blood pressure) to the diet. Go on a 2-week goat's milk mono diet.

CHRONIC KIDNEY PROBLEM

Water Therapy

Follow the same techniques as for acute nephritis. In addition, induce perspiration with detoxification baths, drinks, and packs, and sauna.

Oatstraw baths are excellent for kidney and bladder problems. Immerse body in a warm oatstraw bath for 10 minutes. Conclude with a 1-minute cold bath or quick cold shower.

Frequently apply neutral or cold compresses or packs that have been dipped in oatstraw over the kidneys.

Drink juniper berry tea with a pinch of the herb horsetail.

UREMIA

This is a life-threatening kidney insufficiency.

Water Therapy

Stimulate the kidneys by wrapping the body in a hot blanket pack for 30 minutes. Simultaneously apply a cold compress over the heart. Renew every 10 minutes. Do not allow compress to get warm.

Alternate the above pack with a 30-minute hot enema. A deep enema in the knee-chest position will allow the hot water to flow through a great deal of the colon. Aim for a temperature of 105°F.

This water therapy does not replace proper medical attention and supervision.

PAIN (Colic and Stones)

Water Therapy

Kidney stones irritate the mucous membrane and stimulate the muscles into a contraction. The pain of kidney colic and kidney stone activity is due to the spasmodic contraction of the muscles in the area of the kidneys.

Overcome the pain by applying large hot moist compresses to the kidney area. Also, occasionally immerse the body in full hot baths. During both these applications, place a cold compress on the forehead to avoid blood rushing away from the head.

For intense pain, apply a hot blanket pack or hot trunk pack. Simultaneously apply a cold compress over the heart. Renew compress every 10 minutes.

KNEE INJURIES

Water Therapy

Ice is the initial treatment for a contusion, ligament sprain, laceration, muscle strain, tear, or fracture. Place a piece of clean cotton cloth over the injury and place an ice bag on top of the cloth. Attach with an elastic bandage. Elevate the knee. *If you have a fracture, see a physician.*

General Therapy

Check for *hidden* bleeding in all knee injuries. If you will be engaging in contact sport competition, attach a heavy protective pad of rubber or plastic under your uniform.

Massage torn ligaments with mixture of apple cider vinegar and iodized salt. Overcome stiffness and inflammation with neutral compresses dipped in apple cider vinegar and iodized salt. Apply compress for 10–15 minutes.

CONTUSION

Water Therapy

Apply ice bags immediately, and repeat ice therapy at least twice a day (see above). Continue until the acute signs and symptoms of the bruise subside completely, and a full range of motion is restored.

General Therapy

When the ice is removed, place a *light* foam rubber pad over contusion area and secure with an elastic bandage wrap. The objective is to render light compression to discourage hemorrhage and edema. Use a heavier rubber pad or plastic pad if you engage in contact sports activity.

KNEE SPRAINS

Water Therapy

Use the same therapy as for a contusion—ice, elastic adhesive strapping, felt splints, and elevation of the knee. Use crutches for ambulation.

Cold whirlpool therapy (65°F) helps mild and moderate sprains.

Apply apple cider vinegar and neutral to cold water compresses, or vinegar and iodized salt packs, for 15–20 minutes.

General Therapy

Carefully examine the knee area for blood or lymph fluid escape into the knee tissues. According to Dr. Isao Hirata, Jr., of the University of South Carolina, any fluid escape beyond the second day may conceal cartilage damage.

After the initial ice treatment, Dr. Hirata puts his student athletes on a graduated jogging program. He feels that once motion is possible, proper control decreases the pain in the knee. After each workout, for the remainder of the season, Dr. Hirata applies a fresh supporting adhesive strapping to the knee. In between treatments, he suggests protecting the sprained area with additional foam rubber pad and elastic bandaging.

KNEE BURSITIS

Bursitis is an acute or chronic inflammation of a bursa. Bursa, a word we inherited from the Greeks, means a "wine skin," and is actually a sac or a saclike cavity filled with a viscous fluid and situated at places in the tissues at which friction would otherwise develop. The bursitis may be caused by a single or repeated trauma to the area.

Acute bursitis is characterized by pain, local swelling and tenderness, limited mobility of the affected area, and an escape of the fluid into the surrounding tissue. Due to scant blood supply in the area of joints, this leakage is rarely critical, and is usually absorbed by the skin cells.

Water Therapy

Apply ice bags and elastic bandaging to relieve the swelling. Leave the ice bag on for 20 minutes. Repeat every 6 hours. The bleeding usually subsides in 1–2 days, and another 2 days is needed for the swelling to reduce. Retain the elastic bandaging, and apply additional padding to the knee area in future athletic activities.

Acute cases of bursitis respond to ice massage. Rotate the ice on the skin of the knee until the area responds with pain. Alternate the ice massage with a warm *palming* of the same area. Once the area warms up, massage with ice again. Repeat this sequence 3–4 times.

Just before bedtime, follow the ice massage with 1–2 applications of an ice bandage (frozen wash cloth). The wash cloths will warm up as you use them. Afterward, dry the knee and wrap it in a wool or flannel cloth in order to keep the area warm. Wear pajamas to bed to retain the warmth.

General Therapy

After injury to the area, or swelling from an injury, temporarily cease all athletic activity. The usual recovery period is 1–2 weeks, but the condition may become chronic if you resume activity too soon.

BEHIND THE KNEE CAP (fat pad)

The area behind the knee cap is often bruised in normal sports activities, particularly in the running, jumping, and kicking sports. This pinching of the pad may be visible only as a minor bruise, but stress creates repeated squeezing of the area that may lead to additional bleeding, and a leaking of fluid into the knee cap area.

Water Therapy

An ice bag, ice bandage, or ice massage will help to control bleeding and check swelling.

KNEE CUTS

Cuts, particularly deep lacerations, are quite painful in the knee area. Because of the dead space in the knee (and the elbow), the area is more susceptible to secondary infection.

Water Therapy

Cleanse and irrigate the cut, and apply a local pressure dressing without drainage.

General Therapy

Cuts respond well to the following herbal preparations: calendula lotion, calendula tincture (diluted), or the pure juice of the pot marigold, *Succus calendula*. Diluted Saint-John's-wort, *Hypericum*, helps in the healing of deep cuts; diluted tincture of Ledum helps with puncture wounds.

KNEE DISLOCATION

Immediate replacement of the knee decreases the pain, swelling, and spasm in the entire area. *See a physician and have an X-ray taken to check for any potential internal injury.*

Water Therapy

Apply an ice bag, pressure bandage, and felt splint for 30 minutes at a time until pain, swelling, and spasm are decreased.

Do not apply any weight to the knee joint. Use crutches for walking.

There is considerable controversy among orthopedists on the necessity and usefulness of knee operations to correct dislocation. Some physicians note that the long-run results of knee operations are negligible.

KNEE JOINT INFLAMMATION (tendonitis, stiffness)

Water Therapy

Edgar Cayce advises applying packs made of apple cider vinegar and iodized salt. Leave packs on for 4–5 hours.

SNAPPING EXTENSION OF THE KNEE

A snapping extension of the knee should be checked by a physician. Often when the knee is flexed, the physician discovers that the muscle that is largely affected is the large muscle of the back of the calf.

Water Therapy

Apply an ice bag, or massage with an ice cube for 10–15 minutes every several hours.

Most athletes are back in action in less than a week, and have no additional knee damage.

KNUCKLES

A human tooth may occasionally create a minor wound on the knuckles during contact sports. Since this area can easily become infected, this injury should *not* be ignored.

Water Therapy

Cleanse the area with soap and water, and make sure the edges of the wound are clean. Do not close this wound. Keep checking the flexibility of the finger(s).

Soak the knuckle in diluted calendula lotion or calendula tincture to keep the wound clean and free of infection.

LARYNGITIS

Water Therapy

Follow the same procedures as for a sore throat (pages 27, 34, 204–205). In addition, apply a large cold compress from the throat to the abdomen to divert blood away from the congested area.

CHRONIC HOARSENESS

Water Therapy

Use *tonic* measures to strengthen the body. Tread in cold water several times each day. Apply a cold compress to chest area several times a week. Several times a week sit for a few minutes in a cold shallow sit bath.

General Therapy

Check for the possibility of tooth decay or abscess. See a physician. *Tongue exercise:* Roll tongue backwards as far as possible. Unroll tongue, point it, and try to roll it upward toward the tip of the nose.

LIVER

ACUTE INFECTIOUS HEPATITIS

Water Therapy

The following water therapies will speed recovery:
Drink liberal quantities of hot lemonade or other fruit juices.
Apply alternate 1-minute hot moist compresses and 5-minute cold

compresses to the liver area. Repeat this sequence for 1 hour. Repeat every 6 hours, or 3 times a day.

Take an enema three times a day.

Water therapy, however, does not replace proper medical supervision and treatment of hepatitis.

General Therapy

Pay strict attention to hygiene, as the blood and feces of persons with hepatitis must be considered infectious.

CHRONIC HEPATITIS

Water Therapy

To restore tone to the liver area, apply a cold abdominal compress every night for several weeks. Afterward, repeat treatment for 1 week of every month for 6 months or longer.

ITCHING

Water Therapy

Hepatitis can produce severe itching. Apply a cold compress to the head and take frequent full hot baths. Start with water at a temperature of 100°F and work up to 105°F. To further relieve the itchiness, add either apple cider vinegar or colloidal oatmeal (Aveeno) to the bathwater.

LIVER CONGESTION

Water Therapy

To eliminate biliousness, apply a cold double abdominal compress each night. This has a heating effect.

For *sluggish* liver, apply a 1-minute hot moist compress alternated with a 5-minute cold compress. Repeat this sequence for 1 hour.

ENLARGEMENT OF LIVER

Water Therapy

After any bath or shower, direct a 15-second alternate hot and cold shower to the liver area.

PASSIVE CONGESTION

Water Therapy

Direct alternate long hot and short cold percussion showers or sprays to the liver area.

CHRONIC CONGESTION

Water Therapy

Direct alternate long hot and short cold percussion showers to the lower part of the breastbone (sternum), and to the kidney area in the back (just above the waistline to either side of the spine).

Apply alternate hot and cold compresses to the same areas.

LUPUS

Water Therapy

According to Kneipp, a fine-blended pulp of fuller's earth and water, gently applied to the lupus area, will absorb, contract, and occasionally heal the skin surface. Fuller's earth can be purchased in the drugstore. "Luvos Earth #2" for compresses is sold by Weleda.

LUMBAGO

Lumbago is a term for a dull aching pain across the lower part of the back and the sides between the ribs and the pelvis.

Water Therapy

Take frequent Scots showers with alternate long hot and short cold streams directed to the area of pain.

Use the following 1-hour treatment: Apply a series of hot moist compresses, renewing the compress every 5–10 minutes or whenever it cools. Conclude with a cold friction massage of the area, kneading and tapping frequently. Cover area, and rest for several hours. Repeat whenever necessary.

MALARIA
(Chronic)

Water Therapy

To tone the body, take frequent alternate long hot and short cold showers directed to the *spine and legs.* Follow with alternate long hot and very short cold fan showers directed to the spleen (near the liver).

MASTOIDITIS

Mastoiditis is an acute or chronic inflammation of bone and cells of the mastoid—the area behind the ear lobe. It is usually the direct result of a middle ear infection.

See a physician immediately. Use water therapy in an emergency.

Water Therapy

Infants and young children: For small infants and very young children, apply an ice bag or preferably a coil arrangement with continuous ice water. Place over the mastoid bone behind the ear.

This therapy *cannot* be used for older children or adults as the ice causes too much pain.

Older children and adults: The following water therapy relieves the pain by inhibiting the flow of blood in the mastoid, and by *diverting* blood from the inflamed area.

Apply a moist hot compress to the mastoid bone. At the same time, take a hot leg bath and place an ice bag on the carotid artery (on the neck) on the same side as the pain.

Continue the treatment for 20–30 minutes up to an hour.

Follow this treatment with a cold, vigorous friction massage of the limbs and trunk of the body.

MEASLES

Water Therapy

Wrap the child in a shirt or a towel that has been dipped in warm hayflower tea, and then completely wrap the child in a large flannel blanket. The double hayflower compress acts like a magnet to draw out internal impurities, and brings the eruptions to the surface of the skin.

Immerse the child in frequent tepid baths (90°F–92°F).

In between these two treatments, apply a cold single abdominal compress. Renew every 30 minutes, or whenever the compress becomes warm.

If there is a *bronchial irritation,* add a triangular cold double compress around the neck. Dip the first compress in apple cider vinegar (or plain cold water). Apply snugly around the neck. Attach a dry kerchief over the wet one.

General Therapy

Keep the child isolated for 10 days after the measles rash appears (7 days for the German measles). After this time, the child should return to normal.

The incubation period of measles is 10 days (17 days for German measles).

MENSTRUATION

PAINFUL PERIOD

Water Therapy

To prevent a painful period: Every day for several months irrigate the colon with an enema in the knee-chest position. This position is also soothing and may be used as a normalizing exercise.

Every day for a week before the period, and also 2 or 3 times on the first day of the period, take a brief hot shallow bath. Continue this procedure for several months until you achieve a normal menstruation with little or no pain.

Every morning on arising, drink 2 glasses of cold water. This will overcome any tendency to constipation, one of several possible reasons for continued pain or profuse bleeding.

For the pain: Drink hot herbal teas such as chamomile, peppermint, or linden frequently. Japanese women often drink a mixture called Two Peony Tea. This is available in Japanese food stores in large cities.

Roast 2 cups of rock salt or coarse salt for 15 minutes, wrap in a towel, and apply to the abdomen and ovary area.

Sit in a cold shallow bath and at the same time immerse the feet in hot water.

Apply hot moist compresses to spine and/or abdomen.

At bedtime on the first night of the period, apply a half-full hot water bottle to the area of pain, then go to sleep.

General Therapy

Add additional vitamin C and calcium (both bone meal and dolomite) and vitamin D in low dosage to the diet. On the first day of the period, prevent cramps by taking 1–2 calcium tablets every hour.

PROFUSE MENSTRUATION

Water Therapy

Before the period starts, take frequent hot shallow sit baths, drink cold water every morning before breakfast, and take frequent enemas.

On the *first day* of the period, do *not* take hot baths, but three times during the day drink a half cup of black bean juice. This will eventually lessen the profuse flow. To decrease the flow *just before and during* the period, sit in cold shallow baths. If possible, simultaneously immerse the feet in a hot foot bath.

Sometimes, profuse menses responds to the reflex action of a cold foot bath. Also, you can apply an ice bag between the thighs to decrease the flow.

NERVOUSNESS DURING PERIOD (see also Nervousness)

Water Therapy

Frequently sponge or immerse breasts, abdomen, hands, or feet in cold water.

Drink chamomile or linden tea before and during menstruation. These are calming teas.

General Therapy

Investigate the possibility of occasionally using the herb *valerian*. (See Resource List.)

DELAYED, SUPPRESSED, OR SCANTY PERIOD

Water Therapy

Lack of period is due to a faulty blood supply, which in turn may be due to any number of reasons. A daily enema before sleep and drinking copious amounts of water will stimulate the body to more normal functioning.

Several days before period is expected: Immerse the body in alternate hot and cold shallow sit baths, or apply alternate hot and cold compresses to the pelvic area.

Irrigate the vaginal area with alternate hot and cold vaginal douches.

Apply prolonged hot moist compresses to the pelvic area.

Before going to bed, take a hot shallow sit bath. When you are in bed, keep your feet warm by applying a hot water bottle.

Drink hot herbal teas such as rosemary, sage, chamomile, lady's mantle, or lemon vebena to stimulate the onset of the period.

MENOPAUSE

Water Therapy

Use all possible tonic and friction procedures to increase the tone and circulation of the body.

As often as possible during the day—especially the first thing in the morning and the very last thing at night—tread in cold water. Gradually increase your tolerance to the cold, and kneel in the water, and whenever you can, briefly sit in the cold water. This will increase your energy and zest for life.

Drink calming chamomile and/or linden tea or ginseng powder tea to normalize the body. Ginseng is energizing, too.

General Therapy

Wear cotton nightgowns with no sleeves. Imagine cool places and refreshing water activities when the flushes or the night sweats bother you. During stressful periods, occasionally use a valerian herb discote.

Investigate the Bach Flower Remedies for natural control of up and down emotional feelings. See Resource List.

Do lots of exercise and keep very busy, preferably doing things you enjoy. Add vitamins E, C, B complex, and A. Also add kelp, calcium, PABA, pantothenic acid, hydrochloride, and betaine or pepsin to the diet.

Vitamin E—up to 1,000 I.U. daily; C—up to 3,000 mg daily; A—up to 50,000 I.U. daily; strong B complex; B_6—up to 100 mg daily; B_1—up to 100 mg daily; PABA—up to 100 I.U. daily; calcium—2–4 bonemeal tablets daily; hydrochloride and betaine or pepsin—one with each meal; kelp tablets—several daily; pantothenic acid—up to 100 mg daily.

MUMPS

Water Therapy

Apply an ice compress over the swelling, and renew every 5 minutes to inhibit the spread of the infection.

When swelling is checked, apply alternate 15-minute hot moist compresses and 5-minute cold compresses. This helps to restore normal circulation to the area. Adding rosemary tea to the compress water helps alleviate feelings of pressure.

Several times a day place the child in a tepid (90°F) bath for 20 minutes. To avoid a chill, keep the top of the child's body covered with a dry towel. Dry the child immediately and thoroughly, and put him back to bed.

General Therapy

Isolate the child until the swelling goes down. It usually takes 8 days for the child to resume normal activity. The incubation period for mumps is 17–18 days.

MUSCLES

CRAMPS

Water Therapy

Hand cramps: Immerse hands in *hot hand baths* for cramps due to tennis, typing, piano playing, writing, ham radio work, potting, painting, gardening, drafts, or factory work.

Leg cramps: Apply hot moist compresses on the legs to relieve pain and increase local circulation.

Or, simultaneously immerse the feet up to the knees in a hot foot bath and apply a hot moist compress to the inner thighs and knees.

Birth cramps: Apply a hot moist compress over the pubis and the area between the vagina and anus to relax uterine tissues during birth activities.

Pregnancy Cramps: Add calcium and B_6 to the diet.

Menstrual Cramps: see "Menstruation."

General Therapy

Most chronic muscle cramps are due to the inability of the body to assimilate certain needed materials, or from a mineral or vitamin deficiency, such as a hydrochloric acid deficiency.

Having enough vitamin E may help alleviate leg cramps. Magnesium, potassium, and the vitamins B_6, C, and D are also important in preventing leg cramps. Add a whole B supplement or brewer's yeast, tea made from licorice, and tea made from ginseng powder or extract to the diet. These are said to increase natural hormones in the body, and *may* help with endocrine imbalance.

ATROPHIED MUSCLES

Water Therapy

Apply alternate hot and cold compresses; direct alternate hot and cold showers to the atrophied muscles; or immerse the atrophied area in alternate hot and cold partial baths.

NAUSEA
(acute attack)

Water Therapy

Apply one ice pack to base of the skull and neck, and simultaneously apply another one over the solar plexus. Leave on for up to 20 minutes.

Peppermint tea, or a few drops of oil of peppermint in hot water, is an effective antinausea aid (and will also help with diarrhea). For this reason, I carry a vial of peppermint on all trips abroad.

Chamomile tea is antispasmodic, as well as a sedative. A few drops of gentian tincture in hot water also controls attacks of faintness and nausea. A teaspoon or a tablespoon of apple cider vinegar in a cup of water will overcome nausea as well.

You may add a tiny amount of grated nutmeg to any of these preparations.

NECK SPASM

Water Therapy

To overcome a neck spasm, take a hot shallow sit bath or a hot foot bath. These baths act on the neck muscles via reflex action. You can also soak the entire body up to the hairline in a long warm or hot bath. While in the bath, apply a cold compress on the forehead.

General Therapy

Rotate the neck slowly in both directions. Breathe deeply and slowly. Try to relax the whole body as well as the neck.

If you have chronic neck spasms, see a chiropractor, osteopath, or Swedish massage therapist.

NERVOUSNESS

Water Therapy

Neutral temperature baths help to dispel nervousness. You can also add chamomile tea to the bathwater and drink chamomile or linden tea.

Preissnitz discovered that when he wrapped his patients in a damp sheet covered with a dry sheet, it created warmth, and the patient usually fell into an immediate calm, peaceful sleep. See "Damp Sheet Pack."

Hot moist compresses applied to the spine have a sedative effect.

Hot foot baths help relax the entire body.

Neutral tub baths or tepid spongings of the body, followed by swift drying, help relieve tension. Hot water bottles at the feet are also effective.

For nervous exhaustion, feebleness, or excess alcoholic reaction: Take a tepid shower, with light spraying and no pressure on the head. Apply a cold compress to the forehead. Then, spray the feet with cold water for 15–20 seconds. End the therapy with a bulletlike stream of cold water directed to spine. Direct water up and down and across spine. Do this for 20–30 seconds.

If your vitality is still low, douse your entire body with tepid water. Cover your body immediately with a large dry sheet, and rub the body through the sheet.

Long-Range Water Therapy (See Strengthening the Body)

NEURALGIA

Neuralgia is an inflammation of a nerve, caused by a circulatory problem of either too much or too little blood in an area. This causes the numbness and pain. Both neuralgia and neuritis respond favorably to water therapy.

Water Therapy

Water therapy fights neuralgia by relieving the pressure by restoring normal circulation, increasing the metabolism of the area, and carrying off uric acid or sodium urate deposits.

Use some form of moist *heat* (hot compresses or baths) and follow with cold tonic procedures. Occasionally, only cold is used, but this is *only* when the area doesn't respond to heat at all. Usually, cold will increase the pain and spasm.

BETWEEN THE SHOULDERS PAIN

Water Therapy

Intercostal pain is relieved by a series of medium-pressure long hot and short cold showers directed from the midline below the ribs to the midline of the navel.

TRIGEMINAL PAIN (skin of face, tongue, teeth, muscles of mastication)

Water Therapy

Use hot air bath or steam room daily. Follow with a cold shower or a cold water spray.

Hot moist cloths will help to *divert* the blood to the skin. Apply for 15 minutes. Then use a cold water and gentle friction rub.

Sometimes keeping either hot water or hot wine in the mouth eases the pain.

Any of the above treatments can be reinforced by the use of an ice bag on the carotid artery (large artery on neck).

SCIATIC NERVE PAIN

I have a vulnerable sciatic nerve. This is the result of my posture, because one side of my body is longer than the other, and I used to continuously compensate for this in my walk, etc. Good chiropractic adjustments and continuous low back exercises have helped to control this problem.

Sometimes, when I feel a tightness in this area, I take a hot bath, and afterward lie down on one of several *frozen bandages* I always keep ready in my freezer. The body is always ready to organize its defenses when extreme hot or cold are used, and before long the area heats up from within and the spasm is eliminated. See page 24.

Water Therapy

To both lessen pain and aid circulation, take alternate long hot, then short cold (Scots) showers. Direct the streams to the sciatic nerve. Or, apply hot moist compresses on the painful area and follow with a cold water spray. Or, take a hot hip or hot half bath (100°F), and conclude with a cold shower or cold friction massage.

To avoid a recurrence of the problem, continue these series of treatments.

General Therapy

Investigate possible causes, which sometimes result from tooth decay, extra teeth, or gouty deposits.

NOSE

Water Therapy

The nose is very responsive to a number of reflex points. Take cold showers or massage with ice on the back of the neck, the face and hands, or the upper spine.

Nose bleed: Hold an ice cube in the hands. You can also apply a cold compress (or ice) on the back of the neck to stop a nosebleed. Or, you can sniff very cold or very hot water into the nose; place crushed ice in the nose; or put either the hands or the feet in either very cold water or ice water for a short time.

PAIN

Water Therapy

Hot: Hot water usually relieves pain and inflammation. See "Inflammation" and "Neuralgia" for specific details. Hot water applications include hot moist compresses; hot foot baths, or full hot baths; showers with hot water directed to the painful area or to the reflex area linked to the pain; partial or full hot blanket packs; and hot water bottles.

Cold: Properly applied cold water can successfully relieve pain. For injuries and to control bleeding, apply an ice bag plus compression. Do this immediately. Check specific details for each injury.

Cold applications must *not* be used on bony inflammations, as in mastoiditis, or in neuralgia. However, ice inhibits blood flow in an area, and, when necessary, an ice bag may be applied to the *nearest artery supplying blood* to the area of pain.

Other cold water treatments for pain include drinking ice water; eating cracked ice; immersing either hand or foot or the lower part of the body in a partial cold bath; and ice compress, cold compress, or frozen bandage, depending on the problem.

Alternate and simultaneous hot and cold: When specifically indicated, both *alternate* hot and cold water, and *simultaneous* hot and cold water, are effective pain treatments.

PALM BRUISE

The fleshy prominence of the palm near the little finger is prone to special bruises. Any such bruise should be carefully monitored, as it can sometimes develop into a small tumor (due to a new growth of blood vessels). Repeated striking, as in stick sports, can result in swelling, twinges of pain, and constriction of the blood to the area. This sometimes feels like needles and pins in the hand. Occasionally, this leads to an impaired sense of touch in the thumb and three fingers, as in carpal tunnel syndrome.

Water Therapy

Take frequent alternate hot and cold arm baths, and alternate hot and cold compresses to increase circulation in the area. Direct alternate hot and cold jet shower streams to the area, and take alternate long hot and short cold showers.

General Therapy

Manual pressure therapy, physiotherapy, chiropractic, or Swedish massage can relieve the pressure due to weakness in palm or wrist.

PELVIC AREA PROBLEMS
(See also Menstruation)

Spasms in Bladder, Rectum, Uterus

Apply prolonged hot moist compresses to the pelvic area to relax the muscles of the bladder, rectum, and uterus. This relieves spasms in these organs and increases menstrual flow. To decrease the flow, sit in a cold shallow bath.

Showers on the shoulder area act by reflex on the pelvic area.

Pelvic Cramps Due to Period

Sit in a cold shallow bath. At the same time, immerse feet in a hot foot bath.

Pelvic Inflammation

Sit in a cold shallow bath. At the same time, immerse feet in a hot foot bath.

Pelvic Congestion

Take a hot foot bath.

Noninflammatory Pelvic Problems

Sit in a hot shallow bath or immerse feet in a hot foot bath.

PERSPIRATION INDUCTION

The human body has a network of 2 million sweat glands and about 6 miles of ducts on the skin. When a disease is present, the ducts do not work as well as they should and need stimulation. This is easily accomplished without drugs by using the simple techniques of water therapy. Water therapy helps to rebalance and normalize body health by rushing unneeded toxins and surplus waste materials out of the body in the form of perspiration. This process also stimulates the kidneys so that they function better, relieves internal congestion, decreases edema, and helps to prepare even the weakest patient for possible cold water therapy.

Water Treatments To Induce Perspiration

Sunbath

Turkish, Russian steamroom bath

Sauna

Full hot bath (herbs optional)

Hot blanket pack—partial or full

Dry pack

Cold damp (or dripping wet)
    sheet compress—partial or full

Hot shower

Hot foot bath, hot leg
    bath

Hot shallow sit bath

Hot moist application
    to spine

Hot water drinking

Hot edema

Steam tent-vaporizer

PERITONITIS
(until the physician arrives)

Inflammation of the peritoneum is attended by abdominal pain and tenderness, constipation, vomiting, and moderate fever.

Water Therapy

Dip a large towel in cold water, and spread it dripping wet over the chest and abdomen. Cover the wet towel with a larger dry towel. Draw the bedclothes over the double compress, and up and around the neck of the patient.

An even more powerful and efficient treatment includes simultaneous applications of ice and heat. Wrap the legs alone, or the legs and hips, in a hot moist compress or pack. At the same time, apply an ice bag or ice compress to the abdomen.

PHLEBITIS

Phlebitis is the inflammation of a vein. The condition is marked by infiltration of the coats of the vein and the formation of a thrombus. The disease is attended by edema, stiffness, and pain in the affected area.

Water Therapy

Early stages: Apply warm moist packs. The limb must be elevated and kept warm. Do not massage.

In the past, resting in bed was generally advised. Now, however, many physicians advise exercise, normal activity, and walking.

Recovery Stage: Apply a hot moist compress, followed *immediately* by a cold compress. Keep the cold in place for a few seconds, *turn it over,* and apply for another 30 seconds. Dry the area, and apply a second hot compress. Repeat this process 3 times. The alternate hot and cold on the limb acts as a mild stimulant and tonic.

Alternate hot and cold foot baths or leg baths can be substituted for the compress application.

Edgar Cayce suggests the addition of hot mullein oil to the hot compresses once a week, particularly if treatment is not progressing well.

When the danger of embolism has passed, begin cold loofah or mitten massages. Massage once a day. Avoid touching the troubled vein during the massage.

When only the edema or restricted blood flow remains, direct alternate hot and cold percussion showers to the area.

Take rosemary baths to increase circulation.

PLEURISY

Acute Attack

The following is the treatment for the *right lung*. Reverse the treatment for the left lung.

Immerse both feet in a hot shallow bath.

Apply a hot moist compress to the right chest, and renew when the compress loses heat. Repeat 4–5 times until pain is relieved.

Apply cold friction massage to every section of the body, *except* the right chest.

Chronic Case

Immerse feet in a hot shallow bath.

Apply a hot moist compress to the right side of the chest.

Direct a no-force rain spray and alternate hot and cold spray on the chest over the area affected.

Follow chest spray with alternate hot and cold jet showers directed to the feet and legs. The hot shower should last 4 minutes; the cold shower 30 seconds. They should be forceful.

PNEUMONIA

Before the discovery of antibiotics, many internationally known physicians used water therapy to treat patients who had contracted either bacterial or nonbacterial forms of this acute infection of the lungs.

The water therapy did not "attack" the pathogenic aspect of the acute infection, but was more a *regeneration of the general metabolic system.* Like the classic Oriental physicians, hydrotherapists have always looked at the body in a holistic manner, and sought to tone the entire body and rebalance the internal energy within the body. This helps nature take over and do most of the healing.

Water treatments for pneumonia, as well as other acute infections, are directed to stimulating the body's immune system, enlarging the scope of skin elimination, breaking up energy blocks in the area of the lungs and elsewhere in the body, and creating tone through circulation.

Because water therapy stimulates the body in an entirely natural way, it undoubtedly hastens the last stage of infection—as in pneumococcal pneumonia when the important "macrophage reaction" takes place. At this time, the mononuclear cells enter the diseased part of the lung and engulf any remaining pneumococci and phagocytize them. They actually eat up the microorganisms, cellular debris, or foreign particles. It is only when this self-healing process is complete that the X-ray will indicate clear lungs.

In pneumonia there is an urgent need for absolute rest, fluid therapy, oxygen therapy (sometimes), and body building water therapy. If desired, after checking the blood and sputum for the exact staph, strep, or bacterial causes, you can use antimicrobial therapy together with the following water treatments. Keep in mind that one strain of pneumonia, caused by the *Haemophilus influenzae,* is resistant to the preferred antibiotic therapy.

Water therapy, however, does not replace the need for proper medical care of pneumonia.

Water Therapy

In addition to drinking liberal amounts of water and other fluids, there are two *essential* water therapies. One is the *criss-cross chest compress.* The other is a thrice-daily series of *cold water friction massages.*

Criss-cross chest compress: Tear a large white sheet into strips. Immerse the strips in cold water, wring out, and apply in criss-cross fashion across the chest and back of the patient. Cover the wet compress with dry strips of *flannel or wool.*

Criss-crossing the cloths allows all portions of the lung to receive the beneficial effect of the cold water. Change the cold strips every 30 minutes, or whenever they become warm and dry. If the patient does *not* react well, change them more often. The bandages may be left on all night when the patient goes to sleep. To maintain the cold temperature throughout the night, add a layer of oiled silk or plastic over the wet compress (underneath the woolen overwrap).

Cold water friction massage: Friction wash each area of the body with cool to cold water. Dry as quickly as possible before going to the next section of the body. Repeat three times a day. This sectional washing was developed by Dr. Gustav Nespor, who determined that each series of massages had the same therapeutic action as an 8-minute cold bath. Many persons with pneumonia like this treatment especially because it overcomes and improves the weakened condition of the body.

If pulse shows weakness: Apply a cold compress to the heart area every 30 minutes.

Expectoration aid: Apply either a hot moist compress or a hot mustard plaster. The compresses act as a counterirritant and break up the congestion by bringing blood to the surface of the skin. This will promote relaxation and increase the discharge of mucus.

Renew the hot compress whenever it cools. Always end this treatment with a brief cold friction massage to restore tonicity of the area. Repeat the entire process every 30 minutes when needed.

These same compresses are also useful in treating bronchitis, asthma of nervous origins, angina pectoris, and other chest conditions.

In treating certain pneumonias, such as bronchial or lobular pneumonia, it is also helpful to use steam vaporizers and to gargle with a combination of hot water and glycerine. Use 4 parts hot water to 1 part glycerine. Drink plenty of water.

Diet: Drink lots of water. The minimum acceptable amount is *2 quarts of cold water* a day. Stick to a fluid diet of fruit juices, broths, milk, yogurt, and buttermilk.

Mouth and gums: It is important to gargle and rinse out the mouth and gums with a hot salt solution several times during the day.

General Therapy

The sick room should be very clean, well ventilated, sunny, and kept at an even temperature, almost on the cool side. The patient should be given a large backrest, in order to change position more readily.

POISON IVY AND POISON OAK

Water Therapy

As soon as possible after exposure to poison ivy, *wash* off the poison with brown laundry soap and warm water. Then rinse and take another sudsy bath. This time, rinse the body with diluted or full-strength apple cider vinegar. This helps to neutralize the poison. Close the eyes, and gently pat the apple cider vinegar over all areas of the face except the eyes.

If you haven't been able to wash off the poisons, and poison ivy eruptions emerge, take frequent warm to neutral baths, adding colloidal oatmeal (Aveeno) or apple cider vinegar to cut down on the itching. Soak the area in both apple cider vinegar and the versatile powder of golden-seal root.

Alternate hot and cold compresses (throw away the cloths afterward), or vigorous alternate hot and cold dousings or showers directed to the affected area, will also relieve the pain and the itching.

General Therapy

Sometimes the poison left on the shoes or clothes can cause eruptive lesions, so wipe the shoes with a tissue, and wash the clothes, but don't handle either excessively.

Two pressure points are helpful in relieving the itchiness. Find the deepest crease in the center of your wrist. Measure two thumb widths down toward your arm and press exactly along the center in line with your longest middle finger. There is a slight depression in this spot. Press the area periodically for a few seconds.

Another good point is on the outside of the little toe on the right foot, about two inches from the edge of the toe. There is an infinitesmal depression here also. Press deeply for a minute or so at a time.

PREGNANCY

Water Therapy

Drink water freely to stimulate the kidneys. Especially drink 2 glasses of cold water every morning before breakfast. After this, gently massage the abdomen for 5 minutes. Continue this throughout the pregnancy, as it will help to regulate the bowels.

Take a warm water shallow bath for 30 minutes every day, at *noon* whenever possible. This helps drain the veins by osmosis and prevent and correct varicose veins.

The easiest method of cleansing during the last stages of pregnancy is to stand in several inches of warm water and take a cool shower.

If there is albumen in the urine, or serious vertigo or dizziness, use a hot dry pack every second or third night. After the sixth month of pregnancy, try to develop a *weekly* sweating routine. Drink a large glass of hot lemonade with honey. Then get into bed, place several hot water bottles on the feet and sides, and envelop yourself in blankets. After an hour the bottles can be taken away and you can sleep for the rest of the night. If you prefer, you may get up to cool off your body with a tepid sponging, change your bedclothes, and go back to bed to sleep.

This weekly process will help eliminate waste materials and relieve the overstrained circulation of the abdominal and pelvic organs.

To avoid a miscarriage, take frequent 2-second cold half baths.

PROSTATITIS
(inflammation of the prostate)

Acute Attack

Both hot and cold water are effective in relieving the pain and inflammation of an acute attack. Use either hot *or* cold, but *not* both.

Hot: Sit in a hot shallow bath (8 inches of water). When possible, add strong chamomile tea to this bathwater, or immerse feet in a hot partial bath.

Cold: Apply an ice bag continuously to the area. Take an enema with cold water.

Chronic Problem

Immediately after the acute stage is over, apply alternate *short* hot moist compresses and cold compresses.

After the acute inflammation has subsided *completely*, institute vigorous alternate hot and cold therapies, particularly the alternate hot and cold perineal spray. Showers directed to this area between the anus and scrotum are exceptionally effective. According to some reports, chronic cases that have resisted all sorts of medication respond readily to this treatment.

Another excellent treatment is the graduated cold shallow bath. These 6-minute baths should start at a temperature of 98°F and over the course of time decrease in temperature to 75°F. Add sea minerals to the water whenever possible.

End *all* of these cold sit baths with an alternate hot and cold perineal spray.

PSORIASIS

Water Therapy

Bathe infrequently and do not use soap.

Use the following two therapies alternately:

1. Brief hot baths (temperature 100°F–102°F). Whenever possible, add large amounts (a pound or more) of table salt, mineral salts, or Dead

Sea salts to the water. Always restore the tone in the blood vessels and muscles by ending each bath session with a short cold shower.

2. Apply a hot wet compress to the affected area. Keep the area *hot* with a dry cloth cover over the compress. Afterward, wash the skin with a short cold spray or a brief cold sponging.

Each day, daub the skin irritation with water that has been saturated with sea salt or real sea water.

Once a week, take either an apple cider vinegar bath (use between one half to one cup of the vinegar) or an ascorbic acid bath with the same amount of crystals.

Bathe in the ocean as often as possible.

General Therapy

Sunshine and ocean air help this problem. Many specialists consider psoriasis to be the result of a liver malfunction, and they suggest using lecithin. Supplementing a diet with lecithin *granules* (more effective), and calcium and vitamin C has helped many patients to control the problem.

Do deep breathing exercises.

Add extra raw fruits, vegetables, seeds, and nuts—especially pumpkin, sesame, and sunflower seeds—to your diet. Use cold-pressed vegetable oils only, and avoid animal fats and processed and refined foods.

RECTAL PROBLEMS

RECTAL IMPACTION

Water Therapy

Massage the abdominal wall in a clockwise fashion to loosen the fecal matter. Also take an enema. Add olive oil to the water in the syringe.

RECTAL STRAINING

Water Therapy

Since pain in the hollow muscular organs of the body is due mainly to contractions of the muscles, any pain from the straining of the rectum (or bladder) is to be relieved with heat.

To overcome the effects of rectal straining, immerse the lower extremities in long hot shallow sit baths. Apply a cold compress to the forehead, so that blood does not rush to the lower part of the body. Before leaving the bath, splash the rectal area with cold water.

A short hot enema and a large hot moist compress applied to the rectal area are additional water therapies for rectal straining.

RECTAL PROLAPSE

Water Therapy

Children: Many children sit on the toilet too long and tend to strain their rectal muscles. This creates a protrusion of the rectal mucosa through the anus. Avoid this situation by not allowing your child to sit on the toilet for a prolonged period of time.

Adults: Apply a cold water genital compress. Remoisten the many-folded cloth or apply a fresh wet sanitary napkin (compress) every 30 minutes for 2 hours. Reapply 4–5 times.

RHEUMATISM
(see Arthritis)

SCARLET FEVER

Water Therapy

Give the child plenty of hot liquids and fruit juices. At the beginning of the treatment, give the child a *little* cinnamon bark tea every hour. Later, give the tea every 2 hours until the temperature drops. Also use this tea as a gargle.

Salt shirts: Add several handfuls of coarse or regular salt to a quart of cold water. Dip a long shirt into the salt solution. Place it on the child. Cover the child with a warm blanket for 1 hour.

Change the shirt to a dry one, and again put the child to bed. *The second shirt will bring out the eruptions.*

If necessary, the salt shirt may be used for a third time. This will bring out any remaining internal toxins.

Instead of the salt-dipped shirt, it is possible to use salt washings. After washing, do not dry but put the child to bed wet under light covers. If the child becomes overheated, sponge the entire body.

At the onset of the disease, wash the child every half hour. Later, wash every 2–3 hours; eventually, wash once or twice a day.

This series of water therapies will bring this difficult infection to a close in only a few days.

If it is not possible to use the salt spongings or salt shirts, use other perspiration-inducing techniques such as hot baths or hot blanket packs. Apply a cold compress on the forehead during these hot treatments.

If the child becomes comatose place him or her in a warm bath and rub the child's spine with ice or wash the child in sections with hot water and a sponge. Use 3 *swift* spongings to each series, and repeat series 4 times a day. In between treatments, apply a cold compress to the forehead and renew every 20 minutes.

If the throat needs to be relaxed, apply alternate 10-minute hot moist compresses and 5-minute cold compresses.

If there is some heart complication, apply a cold compress to the heart area every 15 minutes.

Keep up the warm bath every morning for a week after the crisis has passed. Make sure the child is never chilled.

Water therapy, however, does not replace the need for proper medical care of scarlet fever.

General Therapy

There is usually a 3–7 day incubation period, a week of isolation, and then the patient returns to normal. The use of water therapy can greatly expedite the healing process.

SCIATICA

Sciatica attacks respond to a combination of water therapy, manipulative adjustment, low back exercises, and yoga.

Water Therapy

Apply hot moist compresses to the back and sides of the thigh to divert blood from the nerve to the skin.

To relieve pain, direct an alternate hot and cold spray shower up and down the back of the thigh over the sciatic nerve. This should be followed by very brief cold sponging and hand friction.

Soaking in a hot hip bath (100°F–115°F) for a half hour or more relaxes the body. To restore the tone and overcome the action of so much sustained hot water, follow this bath with a cold shower, cold toweling, or cold friction massage.

General Therapy

To overcome spasms, lie on your back on the floor and do a gentle roll with your right leg and hip to the opposite side. Then reverse the process.

Preventive measures: The following position is extremely relaxing: Lie with your back flat on the floor, with the knees and the legs hooked over a chair or sofa.

SEDENTARY PEOPLE

Water Therapy

To increase the metabolic action of the body, take frequent cold showers. Also, frequently use the Scots shower technique of alternating a hot shower (for several minutes) and a cold shower (for several seconds). This is very bracing and stimulating for the body. Always end with the cold.

SEXUAL DEBILITY

Water Therapy

A cold (50°F–60°F) shallow sit bath, with the feet covered and out of the water, stimulates the pelvic and abdominal areas. The bath can last from 2–5 minutes.

Such baths increase local circulation by causing a slight congestion in the area, and this increased blood supply tones up all the local organs. A cold shower directed to the perineal area between the anus and genital organs is also stimulating.

SHIN INJURIES

BARKED SHIN

Water Therapy

Apply ice immediately to the shin, use elastic bandaging to hold the ice, and elevate the lower leg. Do this for 30 minutes every few hours for 24–48 hours, to prevent secondary phlebitis.

If the area does become inflamed, it will be necessary to go to bed. Then apply hot moist compresses and elevate the lower leg. This will probably clear the inflammation within a week.

General Therapy

Even minor injuries to this area of the lower leg can be painful. Lack of attention to this injury, and forcing athletic activity too soon afterward, can lead to a very serious condition called a thrombus. A thrombus is a collection of blood trapped with cells which can cause an obstruction in blood circulation.

When running activities are resumed, use protective padding.

SHIN SPLINTS

Water Therapy

There is no *specific* water treatment for this condition, but treading in cold water will strengthen the feet and the entire body.

General Therapy

The pain in the area below the knee has been termed shin splints in the general press. It is a chronic problem, but many years ago, Yale trainer O.W. Dayton observed that the reason for this chronic pain was *foot rotation.* "Athletes with shin splints always walk duck-footed!" Dayton observed.

Over the course of many years, Dayton discovered a painless method of correcting the problem. Each day, Dayton strapped the ankles of athletes who rotated their feet, and he reversed the rotation. By taping the foot so that it would be inverted, and by instituting workouts in pigeon-toed steps, most of the Yale athletes overcame the problem within a month.

Today, such rotations are usually brought to the attention of a parent by a pediatrician. When a child is 13 months old or so, an orthopedist can change his or her walk so that the stride will be normal.

SHINGLES
(Herpes Zoster)

Shingles is an acute infection of the central nervous system that is characterized by eruptions and neuralgic pains. It is caused by a virus, and though it may happen to anyone, it is most common in people over fifty. One attack usually confers immunity.

Water Therapy

Splash apple cider vinegar on the eruptions several times a day and take baths with apple cider vinegar and neutral water frequently. You can add the vinegar to a hot bath three times a week.

Rubbing an ice cube along the spinal column, but not over the blisters, will relieve the pain. Have someone massage your back lightly until they discover an area of exceptional tenderness. This area will need pressure therapy. Use ice pressure by *lying on an ice cube* that is encased in a wash cloth, and pressing the area of greatest pain. Do this for a few seconds at a time, and repeat several times. It will provide some relief.

General Therapy

Vitamin B_{12} in massive doses has been used by some physicians with apparently excellent results. In addition, large doses of vitamin C and rutin (part of the C family), calcium, lecithin, vitamin F, and the entire B complex family are needed. If you are using brewer's yeast for vitamin B, check to see whether the Brewer's yeast contains B_{12}. If it doesn't, take it separately.

SHOCK

In an emergency, where no professional medical help is available, use these simultaneous and progressive water therapies.

Water Therapy

Lower the patient's head. One helper should be taking care of the patient's feet, while another applies the heart applications.

WATER THERAPY FOR SHOCK

Feet	Heart
Place patient's feet in hot water (not hot enough to create a burn).	At the same time, use these varied alternating hot and cold applications over the heart:
Even better, apply hot moist leg or feet wrappings to the knees. Cover with light blanket.	First, place a towel covered ice bag over the heart for several minutes. Lift it off. Apply a large 15-second hot moist compress.
As soon as the limbs have been warmed and reddened, rub the limbs with cold mitten friction massage. Use ice water for the wash, and rub vigorously. Dip in the mitts 2–3 times.	Next, rub the chest with a flat smooth piece of ice. Use a quick to-and-fro movement. Wipe the water off with a turkish towel.
Dry the skin with a coarse towel. Cover the patient with a warm dry blanket.	Apply another hot moist compress. Follow with ice. Rub. Repeat the alternate applications 3 times.
Treat the thighs and the arms in the same way.	Unless the shock is very severe, it may not be necessary to repeat these applications for another 30 minutes or so.
	Cover heart area with ice bag encased in thin cloth or towel.

SHOULDER INJURIES

Water Therapy

Several home measures will help to overcome general injury pain in the shoulder area. Initially, apply an ice bag for 20 minutes every several hours for 24 hours after the impact. Also use an arm sling for 24 hours.

Follow the ice and sling treatment with moist heat applications to the injured area. Hot showers are best, but frequent hot moist compresses are also beneficial.

After several days, direct alternate long hot showers and brief cold showers to the injury. This will increase circulation and speed healing.

Olbas lotion, arnica lotion, or wintergreen liniment will relieve some pain.

General Treatment

Severe impact during contact sports can cause painful internal bruises in the shoulder area with consequent tenderness and swelling. For this reason, it is vital to lessen potential impact with shoulder pads that fit well and are close to the body and neck. The jersey must also fit tightly over the shoulder pads to prevent any sliding.

DELTOID STRAIN

Water Therapy

The back and front deltoid strains are treated in the same way. Apply ice to the area of the pain. Then strap the shoulder cap with several narrow adhesive strips that run from the top of the shoulder to the upper arm. Over these, place additional strips that run in the direction of the chest to the back, or strips that run in armband style. Elevate the injury with a sling. Reapply ice periodically for 24 hours.

After a day or two—depending on the severity of the injury—switch to hot shower therapy. Continue for several days. In order to increase the elasticity of the tissues and aid mobility, Dr. Vincent Di Stephano, orthopedic specialist and team physician for the Philadelphia Eagles, prefers to use heat, especially moist heat, at this point prior to motion exercises. He then uses whirlpool therapy or hot showers directed to the injured part.

DELTOID BURSITIS

Water Therapy

Apply ice bags and elastic bandaging to relieve the swelling. If there is internal bleeding, it takes 1–2 days to subside, and about 2 more days for the swelling to be reduced.

Just as with knee bursitis, acute cases respond to ice massage. Rotate the ice on the painful area until you are uncomfortable, and alternate the ice massage with warm palming of the muscle. Repeat several times.

Frozen or ice bandages are useful at this time. Apply these bandages in a series of two, prior to bedtime. Dry the area well, and attach a flannel cloth or wear a flannel shirt to keep the muscle warm.

General Therapy

Until pain and tenderness have subsided, keep arm rested in a sling (except during a graduated program of exercises).

SHOULDER DISLOCATION

Water Therapy

No water therapy will prevent or cure this problem, but frequent alternate long hot showers and brief cold showers will increase the *tone* and *circulation* of the shoulder area.

General Therapy

Dislocation is quite frequent in contact sports because of the shallowness of the shoulder area. The best remedy is for an expert to immediately replace the bone.

Relief can be instantaneous if the expert's foot-in-the-armpit traction is utilized.

After the first dislocation, the shoulder can have a tendency to slip out again. Even simple activities, such as shampooing, can push out the round knob at the upper end of the arm bone.

LOOSE SHOULDER

Water Therapy

Alternate long hot showers and brief cold showers to the shoulder area will increase the total muscle tone and vitality. Hot moist compresses will relieve pain.

General Therapy

A loose shoulder can develop from repeated impact during wrestling or football.

SHOULDER SEPARATION (POINTER)

Water Therapy

Apply an ice bag for 30 minutes several times a day. Strap the shoulder cap (see page 198) and elevate the arm in a sling for several days.

After 2 days, direct hot showers to the area of injury. Whirlpool therapy is also used by William E. "Pinky" Newell of Purdue University.

A gradual exercise program should be started at this time and continued until there is a full range of movement in the shoulder.

General Therapy

The athlete may return to competition in about 6 days after the initial water treatments. Add additional protective padding to the shoulder area.

General Therapy

Minor separations are relieved by water therapy and a sling. Major separations of a few millimeters or more must be rigidly strapped.

GENERAL RELAXING

Water Therapy

Take warm baths. Sit deep in the bath with the water up to your neck. Place a light hand towel on the shoulders to reinforce the water action. Rotate each shoulder forward and back. Do slow neck rolls to relax the neck.

If the neck is very tense, apply a warm compress around the neck while in the bath. A hydrocallator hot neck pack can be used. These silica-gel aids retain heat (or cold). They are available in most drug stores.

GENERAL PAIN

Water Therapy

Shoulder pain *may* mean there is an imbalance in the gall bladder or liver. To reach the liver area and increase its activity, direct a short cold shower to the lower right chest and abdomen, and directly over the liver area.

To relax the muscles of the bile duct and gall bladder, apply a large hot moist compress or a hot pack to the trunk of the body. This may relieve the pain if it is due to a spasm of these muscles.

An alternate long hot and short cold (Scots) shower directed from the midline of the ribs to the midline of the abdomen relieves shoulder and intercostal pain.

The following herbal poultices are also useful: hot moistened flax-seed, cooked marshmallow roots, cooked hot comfrey roots, moistened comfrey leaves, and ginger root tea. Place any of these in a handkerchief, light kitchen towel, or cloth, and apply to the area of pain.

SINUS INFECTION

Water Therapy for *Acute* Attack

Vaporizer steam helps to open the nasal passages. Apply Olbas oil or ointment to the nose and sinus area, and also apply hot moist compresses or a hot water bottle over the forehead and the sinus area. This will lessen the pain.

Cleanse the nasal passages by sniffing a salt solution, or use a pulsating nasal spray (see Resources List, page 230).

Edgar Cayce recommended glyco-thymoline packs. Soak absorbent cotton in hot glyco-thymoline and apply to the sinus and nose area. Keep the pack warm with an electric heating pad.

Long-Range Water Therapy

To detoxify the nose, take frequent hot mineral or salt baths. Apply a cold compress to the forehead during the bath. If possible, use a sauna once a week. Follow the bath or sauna with a vigorous cold friction massage, cold plunge, etc.

Start a program of cold water treading, and frequent application of cold water to the body.

Chronic Sinus Headaches

Make sure to keep the air moist, especially during the dry winter months. Buy and use several small humidifiers.

General Therapy

I once had a lot of sinus attacks. At the suggestion of a nutritionally aware physician, I increased my intake of vitamin A (up to 50,000 units a day and then 100,000 units a day), and immediately my allergy to humidity and rain disappeared. I also drank a glass of fresh carrot juice each day (about 17,000 units of vitamin A). I was on this program for many months. Vitamin C and the *whole range of vitamins* may be necessary. Dr. Roger Williams, the nutrition expert, says that if we are deficient in one vitamin, we may be deficient in all the known nutrients, as all vitamin absorption is interlocked.

SKIN

Water Therapy

For inactivity of the skin: Flush the system by drinking copious quantities of cold water, and flush out the colon with an enema.

Take hot baths to induce perspiration, and baths to detoxify the body.

For itching: Apply apple cider vinegar, bicarbonate of soda, corn starch, or blended oatmeal (or colloidal oatmeal, Aveeno) to the body, and add to the bath. See "Itching."

For chronic skin conditions: No matter where the skin is pouring out its toxic material, *arm baths* will help extract and control the problem. Use either simmered oatstraw or pour boiling water over hayflowers and add to arm and foot baths.

Use the following program: In the early morning, take either a hot 8-minute oatstraw or hayflower foot bath before breakfast. Cool body, dry thoroughly. Before dinner, take a very hot 8-minute arm bath. Cool body, dry arms thoroughly.

General Therapy

Adding lecithin and calcium to the diet helps to control some chronic skin problems. It is important to sunbathe, a few minutes at a time, and work up to an indirect 10–15 minute sunbath. PABA tablets (from the drugstore) are useful for sun sensitive people.

Be a detective when it comes to a sudden new rash. Sometimes new rashes are the results of nerves. Use sedative methods. Sometimes the rash is a result of a new cosmetic, food, soap, or cleaning substance. Think through the problem, eliminate possible allergens, and the rash will often disappear immediately! Add vitamin B to the diet.

SLEEP

Sleep is "nature's soft nurse." Most of us need a good seven or eight hours of sleep a night to enjoy our days. Unfortunately, people get rather desperate when they cannot sleep and often turn to sleep-inducing drugs. But who needs drugs when water therapy is so effective?

Water Therapy

In general, if you are tired and want a good night's sleep, a short or long hot bath (apply a cold compress on the forehead) or a 15-minute neutral bath will so relax the muscles and the bones that there will be a feeling of euphoria and pleasant drowsiness. Gently towel your body dry and go to bed immediately. Turn off the lights, do not watch television, and allow your mind to wander and drift into pleasant thoughts.

Mild case of sleeplessness: Drink some mild, sedative herbal tea such as sage, linden, or chamomile. You may add some bruised cloves to these teas. Or, simmer some cloves (6–8 to a cup of water), allowing some of the water to evaporate so that the tea will be stronger. Then add the clove tea to any of the above herbal teas.

Decongest the head with a brief hot foot bath.

Use a series of three hot compresses on the lower spine. Or, immerse your body in a 15-minute neutral bath. Make sure the bathroom is warm, and to avoid drafts either cover the bath, or, even better, cover your chest and your back with a relatively hot moist towel. This keeps your body warm during the bath. Allow yourself the pleasure of leaning against a rubber pillow or a rubber neck pillow (the kind sold as a travel aid for long trips).

Too much thinking or studying: Concentration or intense thinking sessions can congest the head. Decongest the head with a hot foot bath, and immediately revive the body with a tonic measure such as an alternate hot and cold jet shower to the feet. You can go to sleep after these measures, or follow the procedures for mild sleeplessness.

Chronic insomnia: Drink sedative teas during the day. Eliminate coffee and regular tea.

One hour before bedtime, use a tonic water therapy to revitalize your system and stimulate circulation. Two such methods are cold mitten friction massage and the salt rub massage.

Immediately before going to bed, warm your feet in a hot foot bath.

This also helps to quiet the brain by eliminating any congestion in the head. Next, use a sedative water treatment such as the neutral or warm full bath, or apply a series of three hot compresses to the lower spine.

The combination of the tonic treatment and the sedative-before-bed treatment should be continued for several months to overcome the pattern of insomnia.

General Therapy

There are many imaginative exercises that will help you to overcome the tendency to worry and think just as you want to go to sleep.

Two favorite and effective methods are these: Count backwards from 10–1. Imagine you are in some physically beautiful place, a place you would like to return to. Wander around in that place in your mind, and let your body and mind drift slowly into that first stage of sleep.

The second method is: Imagine a blackboard. Imagine yourself writing the number 100 with chalk. Take an eraser and erase the number. Write 99. Erase it. Count on backward as far as you have to go. Concentrate on the numbers. Fairly soon you should be fast asleep.

SNAKEBITE

There is a new antisnakebite kit on the market, and it includes a vital cold pack to decrease the flow of venom. The newest method of snakebite control no longer uses the old criss-cross cut, or slash and suck technique. It is now thought that this cutting technique causes too many serious cuts and consequent infections, and it may also damage muscle fiber or nerve tissue. When in snake country, carry this *freeze kit.*

Water Therapy

Apply a constricting band below and above the bite *without* stopping the blood supply. Restricting the blood flow retards the swelling and spread of the venom to the nearby tissues.

Apply the chemical cold pack, or crushed ice, or immerse the affected part in really cold water. Some African tribes paint a mud or clay "band" on the arm or limb above and below the site of the bite. This acts to absorb and stop the flow of poison.

Take the dead snake with you, and rush to the nearest hospital. (When the snake is identified, an antidote can be obtained.)

General Therapy

Dr. Thomas G. Glass, Jr., writing in the *Journal of the American Medical Association,* notes, "Cross-cuts are totally *ineffective* in severe bites, and damage the tissues in minor bites. It is poor judgment to ask a layman to perform a procedure on a human that he is ill prepared to perform and reluctant to do . . . , especially since 30% of the people bitten by poisonous snakes are *not* injected with their poison."

Obtain Dr. Glass's manual on snakebite by sending a check for $1.31

to Snakebite First Aid, 8711 Village Drive, Suite 112, San Antonio, TX 78217. He recommends a snakebite freeze kit available from Amerex Laboratories, P.O. Box 32827, San Antonio, TX 78216. Cost: $10.98.

There are a number of other instant ice bags that need no chilling, but they may not be as cold as the Amerex one.

SOLAR PLEXUS BLOW

Water Therapy

After the game, before going to sleep, relax in a long warm epsom salt, mineral salt, table salt, or pine salt bath. End the bath with a cold friction massage.

Thereafter, direct alternate hot and cold shower streams from the midline under the breastbone to the navel to help circulation. Whenever possible, use cold water therapies, especially cold water treading, to reestablish body tone and energy.

General Treatment

An athlete who has been hit in the solar plexus develops an acute hunger for air and finds breathing difficult. Recovery from such a blow takes only a few minutes if the athlete is encouraged to relax and breathe rhythmically.

SORE THROAT

Water Therapy

Moderate sore throat: A sore throat is a symptom, not a disease. Use the cold double throat compress or the apple cider vinegar-dipped double throat compress (or triangular compress). The double throat compress is nothing short of fantastic for drawing out the toxins and warming the throat. Renew the compress as soon as it gets warm.

Gargle with salt and water, apple cider vinegar and water, or sherry wine with nutmeg, cinnamon, and caraway added.

Severe sore throat: Take away the congestion from the throat by a combination of reflex and depletion techniques.

1. Soak cloths in apple cider vinegar and wind around the feet. Soon the feet will feel very hot, as the bandage draws blood from the throat to the feet.

2. Soak a cloth that has been folded several times in apple cider vinegar, wring out thoroughly, and apply to abdomen. Renew as soon as it gets warm. This is important, as when the compress gets hot, the blood will again flow in the direction of the throat and the inflammation will return.

This compress reinforces the action of drawing the blood away from the throat and thus decreases the inflammation, and it also increases the extraction of toxic material.

3. Soak a cloth in cold water, wring it out thoroughly, and apply to the neck. Renew as soon as it becomes warm. Be sure to keep the water from dripping on the chest. Also, keep the rest of the body covered and protected.

SPASMS
(see Colic, Pain, Neuralgia)

SPERMATORRHEA
(involuntary discharge of semen)

Water Therapy

To check involuntary loss of semen, direct a 2-minute cold jet spray on the soles of the feet. Do this daily.

Rest the base of the skull on a bag of crushed ice and rock salt for a prolonged time. This inhibits activity in the genital area.

Note: Short applications of ice will, by reflex action, stimulate the sexual organs. Also, consider using a genital compress.

SPINAL CONGESTION

Water Therapy

Apply a large hot moist compress to the entire spine, over the width of the back. This compress diverts the blood from the spinal arteries into the intercostal and lumbar arteries.

SPLEEN
(enlarged)

Water Therapy

When the spleen becomes enlarged, drink up to a gallon a day of liquids, including fruit juices.

For enlarged liver or spleen, apply an alternate 10-minute hot compress and 1-minute cold compress to the area.

Also, take frequent cold shallow baths. Use a simultaneous spinal friction rub (with towel or bath brush).

Use both these treatments *between attacks* to help overcome later infection in the organ.

STINGS

Water Therapy

If you are outdoors, add water or spit to some earth and apply this "mud" to the sting. If you are at home, make a small amount of paste with fuller's earth, apple cider vinegar, and water. This is a heat-and-pain-extracting pack. Apply and leave on for a few minutes. Rinse off with warm water.

If fever sets in, use a series of sectional cold friction massage treatments.

If you are having a severe reaction, see a physician immediately.

STITCH

A stitch is an acute pain, usually on the right side. It is disabling because it is virtually impossible to breathe properly for several minutes during this kind of attack.

One of the most effective ways of regaining mobility is to lie down with upraised arms and rest for 10–15 minutes. If it occurs during a sports activity, the athlete can then return to competition. Such attacks rarely return for at least a few weeks, if at all.

Water Therapy

Apply a single cold abdominal compress to tone the abdominal organs and overcome gas in the colon or stomach. Direct alternate hot and cold showers to the area from the midline under the breastbone to the navel. Tone up the heart area with occasional cold compresses. Tread in cold water to increase circulation throughout the system and to tone the entire body.

General Therapy

The cause of the stitch is not actually known, but several theories speculate on these possible causes: gas in the colon, gas in the stomach, or a brief swelling of the liver from a temporary heart insufficiency.

STOMACH
(see also Digestive Problems)

Water Therapy

Children: Make a tea of bruised fennel seeds. Strain out the seeds, add honey, and simmer together. Give ½ teaspoon, 4–5 times a day, to strengthen the stomach.

Give chamomile tea as an antispasmodic.

If the stomach is in a spasm from overcold drinks, wrap the child in a towel that has been dipped in half vinegar, half cold water. Apply from the armpits to the knees for 1½ hours. Cover the child with a light towel *and* light blanket during application. Use cold water for the towel if there is intense heat, and warm water if the child is shivering.

STOMACH CANCER

Water Therapy

Practicing hydrotherapists report there may be pain relief by applying an ice bag or ice compress over the stomach and over the corresponding area of the spine. The ice relieves the intense burning pain by inhibition.

Dr. William Dieffenbach suggests crushing and swallowing ice to quiet the gastric mucous membrane.

Water therapy does not replace proper treatment by a physician.

STRENGTHENING THE BODY

Water Therapy

Cold water helps to restore strength and invigorate the body. When cold water is applied to only one section of the body at a time, it restores health, creates tone, overcomes energy blocks, and creates new circulation patterns.

Treading in cold water: Start with a 1-minute walk, and work up to a 5-minute walk. Walk in water that is up to the knees. Cold water treading influences the entire body: It strengthens the system, activates the kidneys, the bowels, and the bladder, facilitates breathing, and eliminates flatulence.

Simultaneous arm and foot bath: This is a little tricky to arrange, but I've done it by standing in the bathtub, and leaning over to the sink for the arm bath. Or, you might use a container for the feet, and a container on a table for the arm bath. Use cold water for both baths.

This bath strengthens the body, and is excellent for the recovery period after a long illness. It can be used by those with a cold hand problem or for minor frostbite. Take the bath for 1 minute. Avoid chilling the body, as it negates the result.

Knee showers: Warm the body in a bath, or with a shower, and then direct a cold water shower to the knees at high pressure. This is a very powerful treatment, and should *not* be used for more than 3–4 days. However, should you wish to continue the advantages of this treatment, follow this sequence: direct jet spray to first to knees, then to arms, then to upper body, moving the shower from the knees to other areas of the body.

SUNBURN

MODERATE SUNBURN

Water Therapy

Apply a cold wet compress to the sunburned area and change every hour. Do this for about half a day. This treatment will usually overcome the initial discomfort.

Adding apple cider vinegar to the bathwater, or to a compress, is very effective in alleviating the pain and eliminating the itchiness of the sunburn.

Add colloidal oatmeal (Aveeno) to the bathwater, or use it as a paste on the body. Regular raw oatmeal can be blended into fine particles and used in a similar way. The oatmeal is soothing for the skin, takes away itchiness, and will help with all problems—including poison ivy, poison oak, hives, and allergic reactions—that manifest themselves on the skin.

SEVERE SUNBURN

Water Therapy

Take a warm bath of 100°F, and stay in the bath at this temperature until you feel a sense of relief. An hour in this bath plus an enema brings excellent results. Afterward, lie down under a light blanket to perspire.

SUNSTROKE AND HEATSTROKE

Do not delay treatment. This is an urgent and grave situation. Call a physician if the temperature goes beyond 103°F, and rush to the hospital. If that is impossible for some reason, immediately stimulate the body through the heart and skin.

Water Therapy

The temperature can be reduced with ice therapy and massage. This simultaneously reduces the heat and revitalizes the body. Drench a sheet or blanket in ice water, wrap it around the body, and rub the body through the sheet. You may also massage with ice, but note that ice can paralyze the central nervous system at this time, so a *vigorous* massage is vital for recovery.

As soon as possible, also apply a cold compress to the heart area and cold compresses to the forehead and head to relieve head congestion. Renew these compresses every 15 minutes.

Replace the wet cold sheet as soon as it becomes warm and continue the friction rubbing until the temperature falls to normal or until the doctor arrives.

If the sunstroke occurs outdoors and you are near a house with a hose, spray the body continuously with cold water and continuously massage the entire body for half an hour or more. Also apply a cold wet handkerchief to the forehead.

General Therapy

In the recovery stage, rest in a cool, well-ventilated room with an electric fan blowing. Continue bed rest for several days. Renew cold compresses to the heart and head area every half hour. To restore total normal body functioning, apply a cold abdominal compress, and freshen the compress with cold water every half hour. Avoid subsequent exposure to heat.

SWEATING
(profuse)

Water Therapy

If the profuse perspiration is not from a fever (see "Fever"), use the following two water techniques to help the body to rebalance its heat thermostat and reduce the perspiration:

Apply a cold compress to the head.

Take an alternate long (several minutes) hot jet shower, followed by a short (several seconds) cold jet shower. Conclude the shower with a cold spray on the feet.

TENNIS ELBOW

Water Therapy

For a mild case, soak the elbow in a hot hand bath (105°F–130°F). This has a general warming effect.

Reduce acute inflammation with a minimum 20-minute application of an ice bag or frozen bandage.

General Therapy

The elbow can often be snapped back into place in somewhat the same way a drawer is put back on its glides. Gently stretch the arm out, palm up, and put the elbow back in place.

Several herbal products, such as Olbas oil or ointment, arnica ointment, and wintergreen ointment, may be of help. A new product, Tennis Elbow Cream, is made from the anti-inflammation juice of the aloe vera plant (you may have such a plant in your house). The cream is said to penetrate the skin and sooth sore muscles and pulled ligaments. It is sold in some sporting goods stores and drugstores.

The "Don Joy Warm Up Sleeve" is a stretchable warm up sleeve that gives gentle pressure and some warmth to the area. It comes in three sizes and is also available for the knee and ankle.

TENSION IN HEAD

Water Therapy

Direct a cold percussion shower to the feet.
Drink peppermint tea.

General Therapy

Press the center of each thumb, hand, or foot. Press the upper left side of the skull until you find a painful area. Press until the pain is eliminated.

TESTICLE PROBLEMS
(see Genital Problems)

THIGH INJURIES

CHARLEY HORSE FROM CONTUSION

Heavy impact in the area of the thigh can create massive internal bleeding that can then lead to an almost crippling charley horse.

The player should be pulled from the game immediately. Preventing aggravation of the injury is of primary concern.

Water Therapy

Immediately apply ice packs and elastic bandaging, and elevate the thigh. Two hours later, evaluate the situation. If the thigh is slightly better, continue the treatment for another 48 hours. However, if the pain and the swelling stay at the same level, the case is serious. With a moderate charley horse injury, an athlete may walk on crutches; if it is a severe injury, he or she must be immobilized.

Continue the ice therapy for 30–60 minutes twice a day until the acute signs are gone. Between *each* ice application, apply a foam rubber pad over the bruised area, and attach it with an elastic bandage. This should provide a light tension pressure. Remove the foam rubber when the ice bag is applied.

Under no circumstances apply heat in any form to this bruise. A warm shower is permitted if the ice bag is wrapped over the thigh bruise.

Do not use ice massage on this bruise.

General Therapy

This is a very common injury. Dr. A. Kalenak of Pennsylvania State University notes in *The Physician and Sports Medicine* that this injury is often ignored, especially on the community, high school, and junior college levels where athletes are often told to "run it out," or "suck it up." "This *inappropriate* treatment results in prolonged recovery, and even permanent disability from loss of muscle strength and flexibility."

One way to avoid a charley horse in football is to insist on a properly fitted pants shell in which the protective padding provided for the thigh stays in place.

Once the bleeding stops, Dr. Isao Hirata, Jr., of South Carolina University suggests stretching exercises, heel to buttock exercises, and a gradual walking program working into jogging and running.

If a *massive* charley horse occurs, when the bleeding stops, apply hot moist compresses for a week, and stay off your feet.

HAMSTRING INJURY

Water Therapy

Every 2 hours, apply an ice bag and bandage with plastic so that there is some compression. Leave the ice bag on for 30 minutes. If the muscle goes into a spasm, it may indicate a muscle pull or internal bleeding.

General Therapy

Walk normally after the bleeding stops. Gradually do high knee exercises and jogging. If the bleeding is heavy, delay activity for about 2 weeks.

MIDDLE THIGH

Water Therapy

Apply an ice bag for 20 minutes every few hours.

General Therapy

Place padding in the area of injury and resume activity in about 5 days. Middle thigh (adductor) muscle injury is not too serious.

TOE INJURIES

SPRAIN OF THE BIG TOE

Water Therapy

A big toe sprain responds superficially to an ice bag, elastic bandaging, and elevation of the toe. Soak the entire foot in ice cold apple cider vinegar, or apply apple cider vinegar compresses to reduce the feeling of pain and strain.

General Therapy

This may look like a small injury, but it can keep an athlete on the sidelines for up to 2 weeks. As this is the weight-bearing toe, it must be healed before any athletic activity can resume.

To somewhat reduce the pain, apply arnica lotion to the toe.

SPRAINS OF THE OTHER TOES

Water Therapy

Apply ice as soon as possible for 30 minutes at a time, several times during the day.

General Therapy

All the toes (except the big toe) can be *strapped* to any other healthy toe, and the athlete can go back into action immediately.

STIFF BIG TOE

Water Therapy

Soak the foot in apple cider vinegar or hayflower water. If the stiffness is a result of some infection, take hayflower baths several times a week. Use frequent cold water friction massage on the entire body.

General Therapy

A chronic stiff big toe can be the result of an injury, athletic shoes that are too tight, or may indicate an infection in the teeth or tonsils or elsewhere in the body.

Often physicians encase the foot in a plaster case for 6 weeks, and provide a bar under the sole of the shoe for a few months. The bar allows rocking motion of the foot and this helps the tender joint of the toe.

INGROWN TOENAIL

Water Therapy

Soak the foot with the ingrown nail in hot soap suds for 20 minutes at a time. Use any of the Caswell-Massey soaps (see Resource List) or Castille soap. Cut off the corner of the nail—keep it square—and wrap the toe in a cold compress or cold apple cider vinegar compress. Cover with a dry cloth.

TOOTHACHE

Water Therapy

Relieve the pain of an inflamed tooth by applying a cold compress or an ice bag directly over the affected area. You can also apply an ice bag on the shoulder area on the same side as the pain, or walk in cold water or fresh snow. These latter therapies affect the teeth via reflex action.

Use a hot water bottle to relieve the pain of a toothache that is caused by nerves.

When *neither* cold nor hot seem to work, apply a hot water bottle and an ice bag alternately to the aching area. This often works when single treatments fail!

General Therapy

Consistent toothaches should not be ignored. Practice good preventive dentistry by cleansing the mouth frequently and removing any plaque. Also, use unwaxed dental floss between the teeth. These practices plus proper nutrition and vitamin intake greatly affect the health of the mouth, tooth sockets, and gums, and increase resistance to cavities.

Other toothache aids: Cayenne pepper rubbed on the gums, or rolled up in a ball and placed near the area of the pain, does relieve the pain, as does that old anesthetic herbal standby, clove oil. A cut-up fig laid with the open side on the area of the pain will relieve the ache.

Finger pressure directly under the painful tooth is also quite effective. Use the thumb and index finger and press hard.

Bier system: Still another method was originated by a German surgeon, Karl Augustus Bier, who demonstrated how pressure with rubber bands on fingers can cause a congestion and thus relieve pain, pressure, and congestion in a related reflex area. Today, the concept is sometimes called zone therapy. I use rubber band therapy to overcome a dripping nose at the onset of a cold, to overcome pain in various parts of the body, to relieve eye strain, and so forth. It works very well.

With palms away from the body, lift hands to face. Note the finger or fingers that correspond to the pain or problem for the zone you will want to work on. Thus wisdom teeth will always correspond to ring finger and pinky, front teeth to thumbs, the nose to thumb and index finger, and so on.

Wind a thick rubber band over the knuckle of one of the fingers. Continue winding until there is either minor discomfort, or a bluish, purplish hue to that finger. Then, gently unwind the rubber band and proceed to the next knuckle of the same, or the adjacent, finger. Go back and forth with the winding until the pain lessens or disappears.

TOOTH EXTRACTION

Water and Herbal Therapy

Before the extraction, take a discote of the herb valerian. This is a nonaddictive herbal calmer that is good for emergencies. It was used during the Blitz in World War II to help the British. See Resource List.

Try to have these 3 herbs in the house for this and other emergencies:

Goldenseal (root) powder (health or botanical sources).

Comfrey root tea (health or botanical sources).

Tincture of myrrh (drugstore or botanical sources).

After the extraction, slightly moisten the comfrey tea bag with boiling water. The bag should *not* be soaking wet. Add a *pinch* of goldenseal powder, and a few drops of tincture of myrrh. Apply to the painful area. The goldenseal and the myrrh reduce the bleeding and act as antiseptics. The comfrey reduces the swelling. Occasionally apply an ice bag to the area of the ache.

In an emergency, you can also combine the comfrey with cayenne to reduce the bleeding. However, while the cayenne is very effective in stopping the bleeding, it is also sharp.

TONIC TECHNIQUES

Water Therapy

In increasing order of tonic effect:

1. Wet hand rub
2. Cold mitten friction massage
3. Alternate long hot and short cold sectional (Scots) shower
4. Cold towel rub
5. Pail pour
6. Salt rub before bath
7. Cold shower

The following cold showers should be preceded by a warm or hot shower. Start in only one section of the body, such as the feet or legs, and later add the spinal area or chest. Tonic effect is increased by percussion of water.

Wet sheet rub   Shower and bath—cold

Dripping sheet rub   Cold plunge

General tonic: Use alternating long hot and short cold percussion showers directed to the legs, spine, and feet.

To produce a reaction in a person unaccustomed to cold application: Use a hot spray, and then an alternate long hot and very short cold percussion shower directed to the spine and legs simultaneously.

TONSILLITIS

Inflamed tonsils may produce a high fever and a health crisis. It is therefore important to use two different simultaneous water therapies. These procedures will induce perspiration, eliminate toxins from the body and act in a tonic way to increase the vital signs.

Water Therapy

Cover the upper part of the body and apply hot compresses to the legs, or take a hot leg bath. At the same time, apply a hot moist compress to the throat, and several ice bags to the top and sides of the head. To overcome weakness from the several heat applications, also apply an ice bag to heart region.

After the leg bath, or while the hot compresses are on, stay under bedcovers to perspire. After an hour or slightly less, wash the body with tepid water. Avoid chilling. Next, use a cold mitten massage sectional wash to tone the body. (Optional: Use apple cider vinegar and water).

Then apply a double triangular compress that has been dipped in apple cider vinegar to the neck and chest. Also apply an apple cider vinegar double compress from the chin past the ears to the top of the head. Make a slit for the ears. This compress heats the glands near the neck and the ears.

For a tonic effect, occasionally apply an ice bag to the carotid arteries in the neck, for 15 minutes at a time, several times a day.

ULCERS

STOMACH ULCERS

Water Therapy

Bleeding: Apply ice bags over the stomach, and chew tiny bits of cracked ice to control the bleeding.

Anyone suffering from a bleeding ulcer should also be under a physician's care.

Pain: Apply hot moist compresses to gastric and adjacent spinal areas. The heat diminishes activity in the stomach and causes relaxation, and thus lessens the gastric secretion and the spasm. Renew compresses until the pain is relieved.

Apply hot moist compresses to the abdomen and the corresponding vertebrae on the back.

Or, if preferred, take a hot shower with little pressure directed to the area below the ribs or to the navel. Or, an alternate long hot and short cold (Scots) shower to the same area. Apply a cold compress to the forehead. Sometimes this alternate application will relieve the pain when the heat alone does not work.

With a chronic ulcer situation, take frequent neutral arm baths.

General Therapy

Rest is important. Drink raw, freshly made potato juice, a half a glass on an empty stomach several times a day. Use frequent cold mitten friction massage. Exercise, and get fresh air and sunshine. Swedish massage will help increase the total body tone.

VARICOSE VEIN ULCERS

Water Therapy

Sit for a half hour to 2 hours a day in a half sit bath of warm water. Keep a shirt or a towel over the upper part of the body. The chest should not be in contact with the water.

Also, take two hot sage footbaths a day at the onset of the problem and drink a great deal of sage tea.

RECTAL ULCERS

Water Therapy

Relieve the pain by using hot water. Direct a stream of hot water from the anal area upward and conclude with a very brief stream of cold water directed to the same area, or sit in a hot shallow bath.

Hot enemas or hot moist compresses are also effective.

General Therapy

Several bidets are available from hospital rehabilitation sources, and they can be attached to the toilet. See Resource List.

URINATION

INABILITY TO URINATE

During the acute stage of some diseases there may be a dangerous inability to void liquid wastes.

Water Therapy

Take a warm oatstraw bath, or several tepid 25-minute horsetail herb baths. Drink lots of oatstraw, horsetail, juniper berry, or rose hip tea.

Kneipp also recommends a horsetail vapor bath. Place herbs steeped in boiling water under a stool in the bathtub. Sit on the stool with a blanket over the body, and let the herbs penetrate your system, especially the lower extremities.

Another technique is to take a tepid shallow sit bath, with the feet immersed separately in hot water into which mustard powder is dissolved. Rub spine with a towel. After the bath, while lying on your back, rub the abdomen with cold water for several minutes. Conclude with a gentle friction rub over the entire body.

Children: Several times a day immerse the child in a warm oatstraw bath, or wash the child in cold water. (Cold compresses do not work quite as fast, but may be used if preferred.)

Have the child drink nettle or rose hip tea freely.

High fevers, collapse, shock, hemorrhage, dysentery: Take a series of enemas, as this will cause the kidneys to resume functioning. First flushing: take a hot enema adding 1 tablespoon of salt to every quart of water. Second flushing: One hour later, use one pint of hot water. The hot water relieves the colic. Third flushing: follow with a short cold-water flushing. This series of flushings dissolves the mucus and loosens the membranes, and is also useful in pelvic congestions, pelvic inflammations, sciatica, cystitis, and chronic prostatitis.

Infections, diarrhea, colitis: Use cold flushings with enema. After each bowel movement, also flush with cold sterile water, or boiled, cool water.

Water therapy should be used in these situations only as an adjunct to immediate medical care and supervision.

INVOLUNTARY URINATION (Incontinence)

Water Therapy

Strengthen the entire body with these specific and general water treatments.

Direct a jet cold shower stream to the soles of the feet. This is particularly helpful for older people.

Kneipp recommended the following sequence of therapy. Use a different therapy each day.

Two cold half baths for 20 seconds each; neutral shower first to the hip, then to the back; two full neutral baths, ten minutes each. Scrub the entire body in the bath and wear a towel around the shoulders.

Continue this series for a month. Later take several neutral half baths each week.

UTERUS

UTERINE HEMORRHAGE

Water Therapy

Apply a cold compress to inner thighs, vagina, the area between the vagina and anus, and the lower back.

UTERINE CONGESTION

Water Therapy

Direct a prolonged, cold low-pressure fan shower to the chest.

UTERINE INFLAMMATION

Water Therapy

Sit on a stool in the bathtub, separate your knees, and direct a cold, low-pressure fan shower to the area from the navel to the pubic bone. This cold action contracts the uterus, reduces inflammation, and acts on the bladder, uterus, and ovaries via reflex action.

VAGINA
(see also page 102)

VAGINAL SPASMS

Water Therapy

Douche with hot water or hot rosemary tea to relieve the pain and irritation of the spasm. The hot irrigation increases the absorption of inflammatory cellular fluid.

VAGINAL CONGESTION

Water Therapy
Douche with tepid (90°F) water or weak rosemary tea for up to 30 minutes. *Avoid very cold or very hot douches during pregnancy. Cold douches can cause contractions in the uterus.*

VAGINISMUS (Painful spasm of the vagina)

Water Therapy
Douche with hot water and take hot shallow sit baths and frequent hot foot baths. Rosemary tea, chamomile tea may be added to the water.

For additional relief, also occasionally apply ice wrapped in a towel from the shoulder region of the spine to the neck.

VAGINITIS (Inflammation of the vagina)

Water Therapy
Acute inflammation: Apply an ice bag. Take a cold enema.
Chronic inflammation: Direct an alternate long hot and short cold spray to the outside of the area, particularly to the perineum (the area between the vagina and anus).

Use alternate hot and cold enemas to restore tone to the area.
White discharge (trichomonas vaginitis): Apple cider vinegar and water douches help to restore the natural acidity of the area and relieve the burning and itching.

YEAST INFECTION

Water Therapy
Take one to two acidophilus tablets a day with meals. Douche with a liquid made from one acidophilus tablet and water.

In addition, douche with an herbal/acidopholus/apple cider vinegar mixture. Combine a teaspoon of chamomile and powdered goldenseal. Add 2 cups of boiling water, steep for 15 minutes, and strain. Put aside. Simmer 1 tablespoon of comfrey root, and strain. Add 2 tablespoons of witch hazel to 1 cup of the strained material. Add 2 tablespoons of apple cider vinegar. Add 1 liquified acidophilus tablet. Use 2 quarts of water for the douche.

VARICOSE VEINS

Water Therapy
Varicose veins respond to the application of frequent hot sage tea compresses. Make up a strong sage tea. Dip a folded kitchen towel into the tea and apply to the area. Cover with a dry wool or flannel towel. Cover again with a plastic cloth to keep the area warm. Calendula (pot marigold) tea can also be used.

Drink lots of hot sage tea.

Take long hot full baths. Apply a cold compress to the forehead. Follow baths or compresses with a brisk towel rub and then rest in bed. Calendula tea or sage tea can be added to any bath for extra effect.

Pregnant women: A half-hour warm bath before bedtime will relieve the pressure from the veins of the feet of pregnant women.

Direct an alternate long hot, then short cold spray to the legs. Repeat 6 or 7 times.

VOMITING

Water Therapy

The following therapies all help invigorate and strengthen the system and evacuate the toxic material.

Children: If the child is normally strong, dip the child briefly in cold water several times a day. This will dispel the need to vomit.

Two other remedies are helpful: Fold a medium towel in half, dip it into diluted apple cider vinegar and cold water, wring it out thoroughly, and apply to the abdomen. Cover with a larger dry cloth. Renew the compress as soon as it gets warm. Or, follow the same procedure, but do not fold the towel, and wrap the towel around the child from the armpits to the knees. Apply for 1 hour.

Thirst is a problem during vomiting sieges. To quench the thirst, add a tablespoon of honey to a quart of cold water, and feed in spoonful doses every half hour.

Several herb teas are helpful. Use either fennel, wormwood, or century tea, place it in small drops on a sugar cube, and slowly let the cube dissolve in the mouth. A piece of bread may be substituted for the sugar cube.

To overcome shivering attacks, wash the child using a sectional cold mitten friction massage.

Adults: It is important to evacuate the poisons. Do not interfere with vomiting except when it is too persistent or becomes chronic.

See a physician to check the cause of chronic vomiting.

If there is a need to vomit, and the poison is heavy in the stomach, drink a glass or two of warm water, or warm water with a pinch of mustard powder. This acts as an emetic, and clears the system. If the vomiting is due to food poisoning, act quickly to also flush the colon. First take a warm water enema in the knee-chest position. Afterward, take an enema using undiluted, undecaffeinated (pure) coffee.

If the vomiting persists, and you want to control it, apply an ice bag over the stomach area, or to the corresponding area on the spine. Lying with the head on an ice bag for a few minutes also helps. This technique helps check nervous vomiting before athletic games.

For persistent vomiting that has no visible cause, check with a physician, or, in an emergency, apply a cold apple cider vinegar compress to the trunk up to 10 times before each meal, and cover the area with a dry cloth. Wear this compress for a full hour. Eat a light meal. Afterward, friction rub the body with a sectional cold mitten massage.

Tone the abdominal organs by using the cold apple cider vinegar abdominal compress daily.

General Therapy

After food poisoning, rest in bed, and do not eat anything while nausea or vomiting persist. When they cease, eat light fluids, barley or rice water, strained broth, cereal, gruel, or peppermint or chamomile tea with drops of gentian tincture.

VULVA

Water Therapy

When a fall astride the balance beam or parallel bar results in a contusion or laceration, immediately apply an ice pack for 20 minutes, and make sure to rest, as both will minimize the bleeding.

Wash the area with calendula juice *(Succus calendula)* to stop the bleeding. This is a delicate aid and will help healing at the same time.

If there is no laceration, apply calendula ointment for the soothing and healing effect. If this is not available, pat on honey, for it will help reduce the feeling of irritation in the area, and will heal. Honey is also useful for sores in the vulva.

General Therapy

Check any laceration with a physician.

WHIPLASH

Water Therapy

Immediately apply a large towel filled with crushed ice to the back of the neck and to the muscles of the shoulder. Use periodic 30-minute applications. To lessen the strain, apply apple cider vinegar to the neck and shoulders. Add several cups of apple cider vinegar to warm to hot bathwater, apply a steaming hot towel to the neck and shoulders, and sit submerged up to the chin. While in the bath, knead and rotate the neck and shoulders.

Every day for a week, apply cold compresses to the neck and shoulders. Renew the compresses whenever they become warm. Apply for 30–60 minutes at a time.

General Therapy

See a chiropractor or osteopath as soon as possible. If the vertebrae are out of line, a competent practitioner can adjust them back into place. A Swedish massage is also of help in calming the body, reducing tension, and reactivating any blocked energy areas.

SORE WRIST

A sore wrist frequently indicates gripping the racket or bat too hard and/or not warming up sufficiently.

Water Therapy

Apply a hot moist heat compress on the wrist to relieve the spasm. Follow with a gentle cold friction massage on the wrist area.

Plunge the hand up to the elbow in neutral-temperature apple cider vinegar arm baths, and apply frequent apple cider vinegar compresses to the wrist.

Use whirlpool therapy to increase circulation.

WORMS

Water Therapy

Take fresh wormwood leaves and make a tea by pouring 2 cups of boiling water over 1 tablespoon of leaves. If you are using dried leaves, use slightly less.

Take 2 teaspoons of the wormwood tea in the evening before going to bed. The following morning take 2 spoonfuls of the wormwood tea 1 hour before breakfast.

Simmer one tablespoon of honey in 2 pints of water, and add to the above wormwood tea for extra effect.

Often onion juice made in the following way will expel the worms: Put 2 pints of water in a container with a tight lid. Cut up a large onion, and place it in the water. Drink the onion juice on an empty stomach. (To use this therapy, you must fast for 3–4 days. Drink only water and the onion juice during the fast.)

WOUNDS
(see also Bruises, Hemorrhage)

Water Therapy

Wash with horsetail tea and apply horsetail tea compresses, or cleanse the wound with diluted calendula (pot marigold) tincture and water. The fresh juice of the calendula petals is an excellent and quick healer of bleeding wounds. For deep puncture wounds, use diluted tincture of Saint-John's-wort, *Hypericum*.

General Therapy

Lay strips of peeled papaya across an infected wound. This is the South African tribal method. According to British physician Dr. Christopher Rudge, such strips may be used for ulcerated sores of the elderly, or when antibiotics fail.

Calendula ointment, hypericum ointment, and plantain ointment will all help with the later healing process.

For bruises of unbroken skin, apply arnica lotion or ointment, or Olbas ointment. There is nothing better for a painful wound and shock than the homeopathic 6X arnica sugar tablet.

WRITER'S CRAMP
(see also Muscles)

Water Therapy

Direct a percussion shower spray of alternate long hot and then short cold water to the hand.

WRY NECK

Water Therapy

Apply frequent cold compresses to the upper back and neck. Knead, pat, and rub the area until the muscles relax. Sit frequently in warm baths to relax shoulder tension. You should be submerged up to the chin. Occasionally massage the shoulder area, upper back, and back of the neck with ice.

PART IV

Water Therapies
for the '90s

DRINKING WATER

Daily Water Formula

We know we should drink pure water throughout the day. Dr. Norman Shealy[1] offers this water intake formula to meet your daily water requirements and maintain your saliva and urine at the neutral, neither acid nor alkaline, pH of 6.4.

Divide your weight by two to give you the amount of ounces your body needs each day.[2]

Self Test/Water Intake

A self test for whether or not you have taken in enough water is whether or not you pass water several times a day, and the **color of your urine,** which should be a pale, whitish yellow. If you are passing infrequent amounts of dark yellow or clotted urine, you are drinking too little water. Another self test is whether or not you are developing dark circles under the eyes. If the dark circles aren't from lack of sleep or unusual stress, it may well be that your body requires more water. To clear the kidneys and flush the system kidney experts expect the patient to produce a urinary output of two quarts a day. This output requires at least eight glasses of drinking water.

Water Quantity and Blood Pressure

Patients with known high blood pressure often take diuretics to increase their water loss. Oddly, the water loss may be too high in some cases and might lead to minor dehydration. It is advisable to check with your doctor to make certain your fluid intake is adequate and appropriate.

[1] Holos Practice Reports (Vol 1,#3)
[2] To obtain pints divide the ounces by 16. (16 ounces to a pint, two pints to a quart)

Some people, many of them older folks, don't feel thirsty during the day. Too little fluid in the system leads to low blood volume which in turn can contribute to low blood pressure. If you've been told you have low blood pressure, make sure you have an adequate fluid intake. People with low blood pressure sometimes feel woozy and faint when they stand up. To encourage a stronger heart rate, and overcome the dizziness, it helps to quickly stretch, yawn and take deep breaths.

EXERCISE AND DRINKING WATER
Amount to Drink
Vigorous exercise dulls the body's ability to gauge thirst, so do not use thirst as a guide for drinking fluids while exercising. To prevent dehydration, cramps, headaches or lack of coordination, exercisers should drink about two cups of *cold* water about fifteen minutes before exercising, and about a half to a whole cup every fifteen minutes thereafter. Cold drinks are more effective because they leave the stomach more quickly than warm liquids.

Exercising in the Heat
The primary mechanism for maintaining normal body temperature during physical exercise is the evaporation of sweat. Athletes, especially younger athletes who exercise in the heat, are in danger of dehydration. Dehydration brings on the risk of heat cramps, heat exhaustion, and heat stroke. According to D. L. Squire, Division of General Pediatrics, Duke University Medical Center Durham, North Carolina,[3] "The athlete should begin exercises well dehydrated: frequent consumption of cold water during exercise decreases likelihood of significant dehydration. After exercise, the athlete should continue drinking to replace fluid losses . . . cold water remains the preferred choice for fluid replacement during exercise."

Exercising in the Cold
What about drinking water before, during and after average outdoor activities in cold weather? In an informal poll of fifty people most thought that they needed to drink water mainly during hot weather, hardly ever during cold weather. They are wrong. It is possible to get extremely dehydrated in cold weather. Sweating during exercise plus normal cold weather breathing in which you warm and moisturize the air you inhale can produce dehydration. This makes you *feel* colder.

Warm or Cold Drinks in Cold Weather?
Most people will be enticed to warm or hot drinks when they are cold, but U.S. Army research shows that it takes about a quart of hot liquid at a time to produce a slight elevation in body heat. The effect is so fleeting that you sometimes end up feeling a little colder instead of warmer.

[3]Pediatric Clin North Amer (37 (5) p1085–109 Oct 1990

The Army tells its people to drink cold water since it goes through the body faster.

Older Exercisers

A report[4] indicates that older people often forget to drink during exercise even though they may be hot and sweaty. Since the sense of thirst can fade without our realizing it, exercise experts advise older people in particular to drink whether or not they are thirsty.

TO PREVENT DEHYDRATION WHILE EXERCISING

How Much Water	When	Temperature
2 cups	15 minutes before exercising	cold only
½ to 1 cup	every 15 minutes	cold only

BLISTER/BOIL/HERPES ERUPTION

The body gives us continual signals. One such signal, called a prodrome, is a warning of an impending problem. For fever blisters, and herpes eruptions the prodrome sometimes feels like a sharp or mild tingling or a pulling sensation. Train yourself to respond immediately to this warning signal, and promptly apply ice massage to the area of tingling. A high percentage of the time you will be able to halt the eruption.

The same early ice massage works on boils, and foot abrasions that end up as blisters. In the case of a fever blister, if it forms before you can stop it, apply a paste of salt and water.

CARPAL TUNNEL SYNDROME

Some people suffer a long siege of "pins and needles" in their hands as a prelude to a full fledged attacks of carpal tunnel syndrome. Placing your hands under warm or hot running water alleviates some of the pain. Unfortunately, water therapy which is a merciful relief, is not a permanent remedy.

I had a bad attack of carpal tunnel syndrome and was told by an orthopedic surgeon that I had to have wrist surgery to correct the problem. When I told him I first wanted to investigate alternative methods, this young surgeon surprised me by griping, "Well then, don't come back to me when your hand falls off!" I am glad that I kept on searching for a natural cure because I eventually found it. It included the succor of nightly water therapy, applications of TENS (transcutaneous electrical neural stimulator), a machine which calms down pain receptors, and can help put pain "on hold," and three nutrients. The syndrome went into remission and has remained so for ten years.

Here are three nutrients that work so well when used daily: B6, 100 mg 2 times a day (after a month or so you can cut this down to 50 mg

[4]Geriatrics (46 #6:325, '91)

a day); unsaturated fatty acids (I used the Thompson brand capsule, one a day); and about 1000 mg of calcium (the most absorbable is calcium citrate). Most early cases of repetitive motion syndrome and carpal tunnel syndrome will respond to the hot soaks and to the use of the nutrients.

Therapy	What
Water	Hot to warm hand soaks
Physical therapy	TENS application: on palm/fleshy part across from thumb
Vitamin/Mineral	B6
	Unsaturated fatty acids
	Calcium

CHICKEN POX

From the Children's Hospital of Pittsburgh comes this water therapy advice to parents in caring for chicken pox when it strikes. "Give the child comfortable, cool baths several times daily if needed. To decrease itching, add a cup of baking soda, or oatmeal baths like Aveeno. For fever: Encourage your child to drink extra fluids." This report also warns that giving a child aspirin at this point might bring on the possibility of Reye's syndrome. See water therapies for reduction of fever: you rarely need anything else.

Therapy	Function
Water: cool baths	Comfort
Add Aveeno or baking soda	Reduce itch
Drink cool water	Reduce fever

COUGH

So many people purchase expensive cough medicines. Current research has rediscovered the value of water as an effective cough expectorant. Water thins out and makes it easier to cough up secretions. Here hot drinks not only feel good, but work the best. Try the hot lemonade with honey.

Therapy	What	Action
Drinking water	Hot liquids best	Thins secretions

DENTAL WORK

Most people dread even minor dental surgery. For extensive surgery such as an extraction, root canal, or even the drilling for crowns and caps, add drinking water and additional vitamins to your recovery regimen. Drink eight glasses of water each day before and for at least two weeks after the surgery. Greatly increase your intake of vitamin C, and add extra calcium to the diet, either in the form of skim milk or supplements.

A *homeopathic* tip: In *Herbal Medicine* and other works I've written about my admiration for homeopathic arnica as a recovery aid after an injury. The kind you can use to overcome and avoid dental trauma is the tiny sugar pills which are placed under the tongue. I use 6x or 6c, or 9c or 9x, about half an hour before any difficult dental appointments.

Therapy	What	When
Drinking water	8 glasses daily	Before surgery
		Two weeks after surgery
Vitamins	Vitamin C/calcium	Day before/after surgery
Homeopathic arnica	6x/6c/9c 4 pills	½ hour to an hour before surgery

DIABETES

Diabetics are very susceptible to infections and gangrene in their feet. Diabetics are now advised to take daily, warm water foot baths with warm (never hot) soapy water, and to pat, not rub their feet dry.

Therapy	What	Restrictions
Warm, soapy	Foot baths	Pat feet, do not rub dry

DRY MOUTH

In health matters we sometimes miss the obvious solutions. Most of us take a normally damp mouth, easy swallowing, and a facile sense of taste for granted. It is only when the mouth feels continuously too dry that you realize the saliva production has slowed up. Saliva has many important functions: it is essential in chewing, it acts as a purifier and antibacterial substance, it helps to prevent tooth decay. If your mouth feels continuously too dry, sip fluids throughout the day. A friend who had radiation to her mouth highly recommends an OTC artificial saliva called Salivart, and a moisturizing gel, Oralbalance, on her teeth and gums.

An occasionally dry mouth occurs normally, but if you are experiencing continuous problems, and especially if your eyes are also dry, check this problem with your doctor, and meanwhile avoid any drugs that decrease salivary production, such as decongestants and antihistamines.

Therapy	When	Precautions
Sip water	During day/meal	
Salivart	When needed	
Oralbalance	When needed	If both mouth and eyes dry, see doctor

EAR WAX

If you have a bothersome accumulation of ear wax, you can dissolve it by first applying several drops of warm (not hot) oil. A vegetable oil will do, but I prefer mullein oil, obtainable through herbal and homeopathic sources. Secondly, with a bulb syringe (obtainable in any pharmacy) with your head in an upright position, flush your ear with warm water. To drain the water out, turn your head sideways and down.

HEADACHES (Migraine)

Migraine headaches can be devastating. A friend who is a film actress called to ask if I knew of a herbal or water therapy solution to her debilitating migraine attacks.

We devised a simple plan in which she was to use first a *brief* hot shower and then a *brief, but slightly longer* cold shower. She was to do the following on a daily basis: Every day soon after she arose, or on working days two hours before going to work on the set, she would take a short hot shower followed by a brief (a little longer than the hot) cold shower. In addition, if she had a premonition or warning signal of the migraine attack, she was to stop whatever she was doing and immediately take a hot-cold shower in her dressing room. The two showers have an opposite effect, and this both shocks and calms the body and in her case helped to avert attacks. My friend found relief with this approach. After using these procedures for about three months the migraine attacks abated and almost disappeared after a time.

Therapy	When
Alternate hot and cold showers	Every day and immediately after any prior warning of attack

INFLAMMATION OF THE SKIN OF THE LEGS

Stasis dermatitis is a persistent inflammation of the skin of the lower legs with a tendency toward brown pigmentation. It is commonly associated with circulation inefficiency (venous incompetency). In the absence of a physician, you can temporarily treat an acute attack with continuous applications of tap-water compresses. As the inflammation subsides, use the compress less and less. Properly fitted support hose will also lessen the edema.

Therapy	What	When
Compresses	tap water	continuously at acute stage
Support hose		

NIGHTTIME LEG CRAMPS

Nighttime leg cramps can be momentarily disabling. Try warm baths just before bedtime followed by easy, easy stretches of the legs to lessen the attacks.

Therapy	When
Warm baths	Before bedtime
Leg stretches	After bath

SUMMERTIME SKIN

Summertime skin problems are caused by sun, wind, dry heat, heredity, age and excessive washing with harsh drying soaps, all of which lead to a dry skin. Noreen Nicol, dermatology clinical specialist at National Jewish Center for Immunology and Respiratory Medicine in Denver, Colorado, suggests warm showers or warm baths to keep the skin healthy and moist. To help seal in the moisture, she advises patting off the excess water, and immediately applying a natural moisturizer.

Therapy	When	What
Warm showers/baths	As desired	Pat water/seal moisture
		apply moisturizer

SWEATING IT OUT
Hot herb baths, steam room, sauna, hot tub

Sweating it out is good for you. It is a natural cure. All in all, it is amazing how you can relieve headaches and nausea and a general feeling of malaise by simply eliminating toxins through the two million sweat glands we have on our skin. Exercisers like to use saunas and steam rooms because the steam flushes out lactic acid, the cause of stiff muscles and much normal fatigue. Ninety-eight percent of the sweat is water, but the other percentage is toxins such as salt, heavy metals, nicotine, and other chemicals we find in our environment.

You can provide a detoxifying sweat bath at home. Read the information on hayflower, Epsom salts or fennel seed. You can also drink peppermint tea or ginger teas to induce excretion through the skin.

Saunas, Steam Rooms, Hot Tubs

What is the story on public saunas and steam rooms?

The results of a survey conducted by Dr. Edward Press, Professor Emeritus at Oregon Health Sciences University School of Medicine and former Oregon State Public Health Officer, show that deaths from becoming overheated in saunas and from drowning in hot tubs can and do occur. People pass out and sometimes cannot summon help, or they develop abnormal heart rhythms and go into cardiac arrest.

Dr. Press cautions that the air temperature in a sauna should not exceed 80 degrees centigrade (176 degrees F.), nor should the water in a whirlpool exceed 40 degrees centigrade (104 F.). According to Dr. Press those with hypertension and other cardiac conditions and those drinking alcohol or sniffing cocaine are at high risk. Patients with diabetes and epilepsy are particularly at risk and Press advises them not to spend more than five minutes in either a spa or a sauna.

How long should a session in a sauna, steam room or hot tub take? That depends on the person and tolerance to heat. Some people stay in a long time, others like to leave as soon as they start to perspire. Europeans are very knowledgeable about water therapy, and end "sweats" with cold dunks or cool showers. If you prefer to take a warm shower, at least end the shower with cool to moderately cold water.

The precautions: Don't take a hot steamy bath or go into a sauna or steam room or a hot tub for at least one hour after eating. The reason for this limitation is that you need your blood to be circulating near the skin, not in your digestive system. To prevent dehydration, drink a significant amount of water. Try to replace the lost potassium by eating a banana or an orange. Never stay in the sauna or the steam room if you feel the slightest discomfort. If you have hypertension or have heart trouble, *keep out of* the sauna, steam room or whirlpool hot tub. Recent studies have shown that while heat stress from a sauna generally won't cause blood pressure changes in nonhypertensive people, hypertensives on medication may experience a significant drop in blood pressure which may lead to dizziness or fainting. This leads to a faster heartbeat and in some cases has led to a heart attack.

Can you get genital herpes in a steam room or hot tub or on the benches of a sauna? Researchers failed to find live herpes virus in the hot tubs, but they were able to demonstrate that live herpes virus can survive on the tile and plastic surfaces in moist and warm areas.[5] I interviewed a world-famous dermatologist, a specialist in sexually transmitted diseases, who told me that as a result of her work she would

[5]Journal of the American Medical Association (250:3081, 1983)

never go into a public hot tub. "There are too many possibilities for bacterial growth in that intense heat," she confided. A public hot tub which is not scrupulously clean can also spread such bacterial infections as boils and conjunctivitis.

Researchers have also investigated dermatitis outbreaks from public hot tub-whirlpools. According to R. A. Breitenbach of the Department of Academic Family Medicine, Wayne State University School of Medicine, Detroit, low disinfectant levels and inadequate monitoring are clearly a public health concern. He cautions physicians to be on the alert for well-demarcated rashes that may be associated with improperly maintained whirlpools.

In 1989 *Lancet* reported on an outbreak of Legionnaires' disease involving 187 people who had visited a hotel and leisure complex in a village on the west coast of Scotland. Legionnaires' disease, a powerful and sometimes fatal form of pneumonia, was isolated from the whirlpool spa.

TO TOUGHEN THE BODY

I love the cold-water ankle splash. It's a great wakeup routine, and, oddly, it is a remarkable sleep aid if used just before going to bed. And of course cold-water therapy of any kind helps you to mobilize your immune system as well as adapting your body to cold temperatures.

It takes time to get used to this intrepid therapy, so I suggest you start off with a few seconds' splash, and gradually increase the time as you become more tolerant of the cold. You'll not only feel better and sleep better, since this therapy greatly increases circulation, but as the days and the weeks of the winter go on, the cold weather should bother you less and less.

If you think the cold ankle splashes take a lot of courage, can you imagine dousing yourself outdoors with ice-cold water in the wintertime? In a visit to Japan, at 5:30 each morning I watched the neighbors, dressed only in fundoshi, first dousing themselves with pails of cold water then exuberantly scrubbing themselves with a stiff brush. These stalwart Aikido practitioners told me of others who purified and hardened themselves under a waterfall.

URINARY INFECTIONS

I've long been an advocate of both pure water, and cranberry juice for thwarting and fighting urinary infections. Researchers[6] at the Weizmann Institute of Science in Israel now know why this remedy is so effective. They report that cranberries contain a substance which prevents coliform bacteria, the most frequent cause of urinary infections, from attaching themselves to the wall of the bladder.

[6]New England Journal of Medicine (324:1599, '91)

WASHING FOODS TO AVOID PESTICIDES AND BACTERIA

I always rinse my fruits and vegetables, and I often put a few drops of chlorine in a sinkful of water to detoxify and cleanse the food. The summer of '91 proved that even hardy looking fruits like cantaloupes can be contaminated. During that infamous summer there was a diarrhea epidemic which the Centers for Disease Control in Atlanta discovered was due to salmonella-contaminated cantaloupes coming in from Mexico and parts of Texas. Suddenly we were all washing the outer shells of cantaloupes and other melons.

WINTER ITCHING

During the winter, the outdoor cold air, and the internally overheated, and therefore drier air, often produces dry, even itchy skin. I recently had a mild dry itchy feeling on my legs above my ankles. Before I knew it I was scratching away. Time for water therapy, I told myself. I immediately applied a paste of Aveeno colloidal oatmeal and then immersed myself in a short warm (*not hot*) bath, to which I added some more oatmeal. After the bath, I doused the dry, red leg area with full-strength apple cider vinegar. I felt immediate relief. The oatmeal heals, the apple vinegar restores the proper pH to the skin.

RESEARCH WARNINGS REGARDING SOME WATER USE
Aluminum and Water

Ordinary tap water usually contains traces of aluminum. Because the citric acid in orange juice has a potent ability to extract and absorb any aluminum traces, it is not advisable to use tap water to reconstitute orange juice concentrate.[7] There is also a chemical problem if orange juice is used to wash down a buffered aspirin. The two substances bind to form aluminum citrate, which is very easily absorbed by the body.

If you are wondering why aluminum is a problem, we do know that in autopsy the brain of Alzheimer's disease patients have been found to be a toxic mass of aluminum. A recent British study actually connected the amount of aluminum in local water supplies with the incidence of Alzheimer's in the population. While it is true that the verdict isn't in yet on whether the disease is a result of exposure to the metal, or a consequence of the disease itself, it pays to be cautious about aluminum. It does no harm to be aware of possible sources of aluminum leaching: aluminum pots, baking soda, and some brands of antacids which can contain up to 200 times the amounts of aluminum we should consume in an average day.

Craving for Ice

Do you know someone who constantly craves chewing ice? The need to eat ice or such uncommon substances like dirt, starch, clay or paper

[7]Lancet (339:1236, '92)

might reflect an iron deficiency from loss of blood either through excessive menstruation, or some hidden form of internal bleeding.[8]

Douching

Despite the barrage of advertisements to the contrary, current researchers warn women to be wary of chemical douches, especially if they are of childbearing age. Recent reports indicate that too much douching has been associated with life-threatening tubal (ectopic) pregnancies.

Hot Tubs and Pregnancy

Pregnant women should not go into hot tubs, as they must avoid high heat during the first months of pregnancy. High heat, even high fever, can cause the birth of brain-damaged children.[9]

Fertility and Hot Baths

Excess heat impairs fertility because of its effect on the testicles and their sperm-producing powers. Some families have trouble conceiving because the men take hot baths for backaches or relaxation, or they work in hot bakeries or near industrial ovens. Men should avoid very hot baths, hot whirlpools and saunas, even a rubber sweatsuit while trying to conceive. For men whose work is continuously hot and hazardous, urologist, Dr. Adrian Zorgniotti, of New York University School of Medicine has devised a scrotal cooler which is worn like a jockstrap.

Lead in the Water

Pipes in old houses and apartment dwellings often contain lead. Because the water stands all night in contact with the pipes, the first run of tap water in the morning can contain lead. There is a simple way to control this problem. In the morning *run the cold water in the bathroom and the kitchen for a few minutes before using the water.* Repeat this action anytime the water has not been used for several hours. Running the water cleanses out the water that has come in contact with the lead.

Also, if you think there are lead, or lead alloy pipes in your house, never make a baby formula, or a child's meal, or a child's drink with standing water. Always run it for a few minutes. Don't ever use hot tap water for drinking, or children's food preparation. Hot water leaches out the lead faster than cold water.

Swimming Cautions

POOL ALERT—YOUNG WOMEN: Most young women with a light menstrual flow swim throughout their period. Because they leave the tampon in during swimming, it can absorb chlorine. This sometimes

[8]Emergency Medicine (23 #16:73, 1991)
[9]Modern Medicine (60 #11:23, '92 and Journal of the American Medical Association (268:2348, '92)

leads to a *yeast infection* by the end of the summer. To avoid such problems, always change the tampon as soon as you get out of the pool.

Also, upon arriving home take a warm bath with a cup of apple cider vinegar.

Itchy, dry skin: Some people get an itchy, dry skin from the chlorine in the pool water. Always rinse the chlorine off thoroughly. To reduce the dryness and the itch, and replace the acid mantle protection lost through swimming, apply diluted or full strength apple cider vinegar to the body.

Hair: Chlorine in the pool inevitably dries the ends of the hair out. Shampoo and condition your hair as often as possible.

OCEAN ALERT—STINGS: Anyone who swims in the ocean in Florida knows about jellyfish stings. If despite your caution you are stung, soak the affected part in *salt water* and then pack the wound with sand, then wash off again with salt water. Fresh water will not work. When you get home pat the wound with the flesh of a papaya fruit, papaya juice or a papaya-based tenderizer.

USING CLAY WITH WATER AND HERBS FOR SPECIAL HEALING

Keep a pound or two of neutral white or gray clay on hand (ceramic marmalade jugs are useful) for a wide variety of healing actions to alleviate diarrhea, burns, neuritis attacks, swellings, bruises, and some chronic pain. Clay can be used alone or mixed with an herbal oil, or an assortment of herbs for nerve inflammation problems. Clay water and herbal infusions, and heated leaves of cabbage, or raw, grated potato are ideal rotation partners in reducing resistant skin swellings, even minor topical growths, and in lessening some arthritic pain.

Applying Clay Poultices

Clay can be added to either an herbal oil, a strained herbal infusion or decoction, or pure water to prepare a thin paste. Apply the paste directly to the skin, or preferably, because it dries and flakes, on a clean white cloth or wide gauze which can be lifted intact from the problem area. To prevent the clay "peeling," cover the application with thin cloth strips, or loosely with an elastic bandage such as used for sports injuries. Or attach long Velcro straps to bind poultices. The straps are available in some rehabilitation specialty shops.

Chronic Arthritic Pain

For arthritic pain, combine clay and castor oil to produce a healing poultice. Since clay soothes but does not bring circulation to the skin surface, interchange the clay and castor oil poultice with heated and (rib-softened) large cabbage leaf poultices. Cabbage *draws out* toxins (for this reason, it can be used to draw out pus from wounds, too). Other times, to create internal and surface circulation and heat, combine clay paste and tiny amounts of such counterirritant herbs as eucalyptus oil or juniper needle oil. An easy way to produce similar external heat is to combine clay and small quantities of Tiger Balm, an ointment containing five counterirritant herbs. Apply all of these in overnight poultices.

Nerve Inflammation (Neuritis)

Neuritis pain is insidious. Heat applications help. Do not use heating pads because of the danger of electromagnetic rays from these pads. Instead use a combination of hot water compresses, hot water bottle applications, and/or heated herbal compresses. If these don't work, combine clay and a heated *herbal oil* together to produce a thin, gummy paste. The two healing oils that are most effective are castor oil or St. John's wort oil. In a pinch you can use heated olive oil. The oil has four actions here: it provides its own healing power, makes the area feel warm, keeps the clay supple, and in the right combination prevents the clay from drying and flaking. Reinforce the heating action by initially applying a hot water bottle over the poultice. After the hot water bottle cools down, discard it, but keep the poultice on as long as you can, preferably overnight. This can be repeated as often as needed.

The herb *lemon balm* is also effective for neuritis pain. Make the lemon balm into a strong tea, strain, and add as a source of liquid to the clay for a thin poultice application. *Comfrey* liquid can be added to clay poultices to relieve pressure and nerve damage pain. If only the *ointment* of comfrey is available, alternate gentle *topical* applications of the ointment with clay poultices, or any of the clay plus herb poultices.

Diarrhea

Clay pellets or clay diluted in a glass of water are helpful in treating most kinds of diarrhea. Do not take any but the purest clay internally. Add any quieting herbal infusion (tea) to the clay water. Since pure Coca-Cola syrup (or Classic Coke) is especially useful in diarrhea, you can combine a mashed pellet of clay in pure water plus a dollop of Coke syrup. Activated charcoal tablets are also valuable for diarrhea. Like the clay, such tablets absorb the internal toxins causing the diarrhea attack.

Burns

The first, most successful remedy for minor burns is ice water application. But sometimes even when the ice water cleanses the charred area (it becomes clean and white), there is still residual pain which causes throbbing. Add a thin "mask" of clay over the newly healed burn to further heal and shield the area from the air. This absence of air soothes the pain, and influences healing. Since the clay dries and sheds, wind a light layer of gauze over the clay. If the pain persists, apply a fresh dose of wet clay to close it off from the air.

Swellings and Small Growths

Herbs and clays have been used for thousands of years to diminish swellings and some growths. Some success has been reported with the use of castor oil poultices alone, or in combination with clay paste poultices. Several herbs are said to be effective in reducing bumps, swellings and new growths. Add these herbs to clay poultices: either strained horsetail infusion (tea), or an infusion of marigold (calendula) tea, or strained oak bark decoction (simmered "soup" of bark), or blended ground-up bran plus a little water.

Heated organic cabbage leaf poultices can be alternated with the various clay poultices. To lessen possible skin reactions, such as blisters on sensitive skin; before applying the heated and softened cabbage leaf, first pat on a thin layer of oil. Some people may have an initial period of mild pain in response to the powerful, detoxifying cabbage application. The pain will subside.

Raw, grated organic potato poultices can also be used alternately with clay poultices on a variety of bruises, inflammations, slow-healing wounds, and wounds with pus discharges. Combine the grated potato with milk and apply directly to the skin, or use it as a poultice encased in gauze or clean cloth. Depending on one's reaction to cold and heat, potato poultices can be used warm, or cold.

Very resistant swellings often respond to a rotation series of poultices of clay and warm oil, cabbage and then potato. These three actions and sequences can be repeated.

WATER THERAPY FOR THE BABY
Strengthening Your Child

Accustom your child to cold water applications. End every warm bath with seconds of a cold water splash. Work up to a few seconds of just cold water. Later show and share with your child how you walk or stand in cold running water in the bathtub. Keep strict safety precautions by holding on to bar rail. Cold dips, and walking in cold water will have a positive lifelong impact on your child's good health.

Teething

Soak a few clean washcloths in cold water and store each one in a separate plastic bag in the freezer. The frozen cloth makes a good crunchy nibble, and relieves the pain of teething.

Congestion

If your child has a congested nose, keep a steam vaporizer going in her room. If you don't have a vaporizer (get one soon!) turn your bathroom into a sauna by closing the door of the bathroom, and turning on the hot water in the shower (close the curtains so the child won't get splashed). Wrap up your ailing, congested child and let him sit in the steamy bathroom for five minutes or so. Steam unclogs those nasal and sinus passages.

Crying Spell

Do you want to see magic? Gently place a fitful child in a warm bath and the crying should stop. This can be done any time of the day or night.

Sleepless Baby

If the baby can't get to sleep, prepare a warm bath, and let the child soak for a few minutes. Wrap the child in a large towel, put on pj's, cover with light blanket. According to the journal of the American Sleep Disorders Association, the warm bath raises the core body temperature; and the "compensatory cooling down afterwards helps deepen sleep."

Nightmare Zap

Create an instant monster zap machine. Into a plastic spray bottle pour fresh water, green or blue vegetable coloring, and some wonderful spice extract such as vanilla or cinnamon or nutmeg, because monsters don't like 'that' good smell. You and your child, or if old enough, your child alone, sprays under the bed, around the bed, in the closet until all the bogeymen are named and routed.

Blister

Rub emerging blister with ice cube to arrest it.

Bleeding

First wash a cut. To soften the impact of blood flowing try to use a red washcloth. Apply either calendula lotion or calendula succus or Dickinson's triple distilled WITCH HAZEL EXTRACT to stop bleeding from cuts.

Boils

Massage ice on first indication of boil to halt it.

Vomiting or Diarrhea

Prevent dehydration by letting the child suck on crushed ice. For diarrhea, in addition to giving the child small teaspoons of pure Coca-Cola syrup (or Classic Coke) to cure the diarrhea, add teaspoons of the syrup to pure water and freeze as ice cubes. Crush the ice cubes, or place in a clean washcloth so that they can be sucked.

Pains and Bruises

After washing a wound, bruise or sports injury, apply ice pack for twenty minutes of every hour for 24 hours. The ice prevents blood from collecting in and around the bruise or wound. For young children here are some fun and distracting ice applications:

Cat or Dog Washcloth-Icebag Sew two washcloths into the shape of a cat or dog to use as an icebag. Let your youngster name the dog or cat.

Plastic "ice cubes" can be purchased in various colors and shapes in hardware stores or housewares departments. Keep these plastic cubes in net or plastic bag in freezer. Apply to bruises and bumps instead of ordinary ice. Let your child choose the color and shape to distract from the initial shock and pain of the thump.

Stings and Bites

Apply Dickinson's Witch Hazel Extract.

Taking Bad-Tasting Medicine

Many children resist taking liquid medicine. Let the child suck on an ice cube first to numb his mouth, then give the medicine. Another method is to crush ice and put the medicine in the crushed ice and let the child suck on the ice.

Tummyachers

Dilute your favorite herbal teas such as chamomile (don't give to child if she has hayfever), peppermint, linden, fennel. Add half water, half herbal tea.

Cold Sores

At the first indication of an emerging cold sore, rub an ice cube on the area. If you catch it right away, you will halt the eruption.

Appendixes

SPECIAL REFLEX EFFECTS OF SHORT COLD APPLICATIONS

A short, very cold percussion shower directed to a reflex area causes active dilation of the blood vessels in the related viscera.

To Affect These Organs	Use These Short Cold Applications
BRAIN (mental activity)	Short splashes to stimulate the face and head; also cold compresses.
LUNGS	Chest friction, as in cold rub, or douches at first increase respiration. Soon they result in deeper respiration with a somewhat slowed rate.
HEART RATE and FORCE	Cold shower over heart, or slapping chest with cold towel, increases both the heart rate and force. After the end of the application, the rate decreases while the force remains increased.
UTERUS	Short cold shower to the back of hip area or feet causes dilation of the vessels of the uterus.
BLADDER, BOWELS, and UTERUS	Short applications to abdomen, hands, or feet cause contractions of the muscles.
KIDNEY SECRETION (increased)	Short cold douche or ice bag intermittently to the lower third of the breastbone (sternum) increases release of urine.
LIVER	Very short cold shower on liver causes active dilation of its vessels and increases gastric secretion.
GASTROINTESTINAL	Moderately prolonged cold application to the middle abdomen over the navel increases gastric secretion.

SPECIAL REFLEX EFFECTS OF PROLONGED COLD WATER APPLICATIONS

A continuous local application of cold causes contraction of the muscles and decreases the vital activities of the surface, as well as the internal area connected by reflex.

To Affect These Organs	Use These Prolonged Cold Applications
ARTERY	Cold applied over the trunk of an artery causes contraction of the artery and its furthest branches, e.g. ice bags applied over the carotid arteries decrease the blood going to the brain and head.
BRAIN	Prolonged immersion of hands in cold water causes contraction. Long cold applications to the face, forehead, scalp, and back of the neck cause contraction of the blood vessels of the brain.
NASAL MUCOUS MEMBRANE	Prolonged immersion of hands in cold water causes contraction of the vessels of the nasal mucous membranes. *Note:* Holding ice in your hand will overcome a nosebleed.
THYROID	Ice bag over the thyroid decreases its vascularity and lessens its glandular activity.
LUNGS	Long cold applications to the chest contract the vessels of the lungs, slow respiration, and increase its depth.
STOMACH	Ice bag to the area between the navel and ribs causes contraction of the vessels of the stomach. This lessens gastric secretion while application continues.
PELVIS	Long cold applications to the pelvis, groin, or inner surface of the thighs contract the blood vessels of the pelvic organs.
UTERUS	Long cold shallow sit bath causes firm contraction of the uterine muscle. A prolonged cold application to the back area between the hips (sacrum) dilates the blood vessels of the uterus; this increases menstrual flow and decreases pain.
KIDNEY	Ice bag in the lower third of the breastbone (sternum), or in the same area on the back, creates contraction of blood vessels of the kidneys.
THROAT	Ice bag to the side of the neck below the jaw contracts the blood vessels of the pharynx.

REFLEX EFFECTS OF PROLONGED HOT APPLICATIONS
ON FUNCTIONS WITHIN THE BODY

A very prolonged hot application to the reflex area produces passive dilation of the blood vessels of the related organ.

Function	Application/Facilitation
HEART RATE	Long hot applications to the precordia (area around the heart) and to many other parts lower blood pressure.

Table continued on page 244

REFLEX EFFECTS OF PROLONGED HOT APPLICATIONS
ON FUNCTIONS WITHIN THE BODY

Function	Application/Facilitation
RESPIRATION and EXPECTORATION	Hot moist applications to the chest increase respiration and expectoration.
GASTRIC SECRETION (increased)	Long, moderately hot applications over the stomach after meals increase gastric secretion and hasten digestion.
GASTRIC SECRETION (decreased)	Before meals, long moderately hot applications over the stomach decrease secretion. This is due to atonic reaction which ensues.
PERISTALSIS (lessened)	Prolonged hot applications to the abdomen decreases peristalsis, relieves pain of spasms.
INTESTINAL COLIC	Prolonged hot applications relieve pain due to muscle spasm.
BLADDER, RECTUM, UTERUS (increased menstrual flow)	Prolonged hot applications to the pelvis, such as a hot moist compress, hot pack, or shallow sit bath, relax the muscles of these organs, dilate their blood vessels, and relieve spasms in these organs.
KIDNEY or GALL BLADDER COLIC	Large hot applications to the trunk, such as a hot pack, relax the muscles of these organs and aid in relieving pain due to spasms.

ALTERNATE HOT AND COLD
APPLICATIONS TO THE SAME AREA

THERAPEUTIC USES

Acute infections of the hand, arm, or foot—*avoid* massage, friction, or percussion. This spreads the bacteria to other parts of the body.
Convalescence—for local infections.
Liver—chronic congestion.
Pelvic area—chronic congestion as in the uterus, or after an infection.
Menstrual period—when delayed or scanty.
Muscles—when atrophied.
Osteomyelitis—chronic.
Ulcerated varicose veins

Alternate hot and cold applications to the same area cause alternating constriction and dilation. This increases the number of white blood cells in a given part, and so makes this technique valuable in acute congestions and inflammation, particularly in hand and foot infections. The same technique is excellent for chronic congestion.

Types of Alternate Applications to the Same Area

Moist hot compresses, with ice compresses
Alternate hot and cold partial or full body packs
Alternate hot and cold shallow sit bath

Alternate hot and cold foot or leg bath
Alternate hot and cold arm or hand bath
Alternate hot and cold vaginal douche or rectal irrigation

HOT OR COLD OR SIMULTANEOUS HOT AND COLD APPLICATIONS TO DIFFERENT AREAS

With the application of either all cold, or all hot, or simultaneous hot and cold to *different* areas, you can cause a withdrawal of blood from one area (depletion). This causes a shunting of the blood to another area.

When heat is used alone, always end the treatment with cold friction massage with a wash cloth or rough mitten. This helps the area to *maintain* the reaction obtained.

EFFECTS OF COLD AND HEAT ON THE BODY

An application of either moist heat or cold produces a series of internal responses, two of the main ones being *tonic* and its reverse, *atonic*. When there is a tonic reaction, the body feels invigorated, muscles can be used to greater capacity, and there are these body responses: reddened skin, slowed pulse, increased arterial tension, expansion of internal blood vessels, lowering of temperature, increased production of heat, increased skin action, and increased total breathing activity.

An atonic reaction means that there is a lessening of tone in the whole body, or a specific area, a decrease of muscle ability, and a feeling of lassitude. Among the body responses are an increase in the pulse rate, a pale skin, lower temperature, less skin action, less production of air from the lungs, contraction of the blood vessels, and a lessening of heat production.

General Effect of Cold and Heat

On the whole, *heat* sedates, quiets, soothes the body and depresses internal activity. *Cold* acts to stimulate and invigorate the body.

Cold: Cold water depresses vital functions at first, but the body reacts with greatly heightened internal activity.

A short cold application is tonic.

A long cold application is depressant.

Use ice to overcome initial bleeding in wounds or pain caused by spasms. Use ice for 20 minutes, then stop for several hours. See instructions for each specific problem.

Heat: The primary action of heat is excitation, but it then lessens the activity in the body.

A short hot application depresses and depletes the tone. This is an atonic reaction.

A long hot application results in a combined depressant and excitant reaction.

Effect on Skin

Cold: A cold application at first produces less activity, but the reaction causes a secondary *increase* of skin activity, and a lessening of sensitivity. This numbness is useful for injuries. Cold stops bleeding.

Heat: At first there is more activity with a heat application. But the reaction causes less skin activity and less sensitivity. Heat is not to be used in initial stages of an injury as it increases tissue fluids and bleeding.

Effect on the Nerves

Cold: A cold application numbs and paralyzes initially, but the final reaction is tonic, and it results in a vigorous feeling.

Heat: An application of heat first excites the nerves, but the reaction creates a lessening of tone, and the result is depressant. This acts to soothe, quiet, and sedate spasms, and generally relax the entire body. It creates lassitude.

Effect on the Heart

Cold: Cold causes blood vessels to contract. The heart first goes faster, then slows down. There is *increased force* in the heart action, as well as *increased tone and activity.* Cold compresses, or ice bags to the precordia, the heart area, keep the area stable during any heat application.

Heat: Heat causes blood vessels to contract and widen (dilate). The heart action slows down initially, *then gets faster.* There is *less force* and *lowered tone.* While this is useful in some cases, it is generally not advisable to use intense heat because of its effect on the heart.

Effect on the Lungs

Cold: Cold slows and *deepens* respiration. There is an increase in the amount of air breathed in and out, and an increase in the oxygen (O) taken in and the carbon dioxide (CO_2) eliminated.

Heat: Heat increases elimination of carbon dioxide and makes breathing easier, as does breathing in moist air in the form of *steam.* There is a decrease in the amount of air given off.

Effect on Metabolism

Cold: Cold increases the carbon dioxide, and improves cell activity and oxidation. It increases urea excreted through the urine. This is especially true after cold half baths. Cold baths increase the acidity of urine, even the urine of alkaline vegetarian diets.

Heat: Heat decreases carbon dioxide, and decreases the volume of the urine.

The application of heat over a large area diminishes the acidity of the urine, and it may become alkaline.

Effect on Muscles

Cold: A short cold application increases muscle ability and range. A long cold application lessens the muscle capability and response.

Heat: A short hot application reduces muscle fatigue. A long hot application lessens ability and response.

Effect on Blood

Cold: Cold increases the blood count, particularly the leucocytes.
Heat: Heat decreases the number of leucocytes and red blood cells.

Effect on the Kidneys

Cold: Cold congests the area and excites the function.
Heat: Heat lessens activity and takes blood from the area.

Effect on the Stomach

Cold: Cold increases activity and increases production of hydrochloric acid.
Heat: Heat lessens activity and lessens production of hydrochloric acid.

Effect on Production of Heat

Cold: A short cold application increases heat production, while a prolonged cold application lessens heat production.
Heat: A short hot application decreases heat production. Prolonged hot application increases heat production.

RESOURCE LIST

Therapy Products Using Water

Steam Inhaler. Bernhard Steam Inhaler. Bronson Pharmaceuticals, 4426 Rinetti Lane, PO Box 628, La Canada, CA 91012-0628; 1-800-732-3323. The inhaler is only 7½ inches tall, weighs 16 ounces, converts to local voltage anywhere, uses tap water; drugless relief for congestions, colds, sinus, throat and allergy conditions.

Foot Bath/Face Sauna. Attitudes, 1-800-525-2468. Portable foot bath includes reflex massage pad, heat and whirlpool bubbles; face sauna has directed steam for sinus relief, aromatherapy and skin cleansing.

Sitz Bath. Duro-Med, Hackensack, NJ: for local distributor, call 1-800-525-2468. Half-bath for lower extremities.

Humidifier. Portable 4–6 gallon model. Hammacher Schlemmer, 147 East 57th Street, New York, NY 10022; 1-800-283-9400. Claimed to eliminate up to 97% of bacteria found in most mist; also to remove dust, smoke and irritants in air. Demineralizer eliminates white dust residue.

Hot Water Bottle. Hard-to-find British flannel-clad hot water bottle. Vermont Country Store, PO Box 1108, Route 7, North Manchester Center, VT 05255; 802 362-4647. Use instead of electric heating pad.

Home Saunas, Hot Tubs, Whirlpools, Steam Baths

Built-in Sauna Rooms, Steam Rooms, Accessories. Thermasol; (eastern) 1-800-631-1601, (western) 1-800-776-1711.

Hot Tubs, Steam Rooms, Saunas, Whirlpools. Baths and Spas International, 1-800-875-2600.

Portable Whirlpools. Jacuzzi, 1-800-288-4002.

Bath Products

Detoxifying. Hayflower Bath Extract. Biokosma, Switzerland; available at better health stores and from Caswell-Massey (oldest pharmacy in the USA); call 1-800-326-0500 for catalog. Extract of alpine flowers, horse chestnut and juniper for use in bath or compresses.

Mustard Bath. Dr. Singha's Mustard Bath. Natural Therapeutics Centre, 2500 Side Cove, Austin, TX 78704; 512 444-2862. Formulated by Dr. Shyam Singha, a London acupuncturist and naturopath, this is made of

powder from English mustard seeds and essential oils of eucalyptus, rosemary, wintergreen and thyme; function is to stimulate circulation and relieve aches and pains of cold; best used as a foot bath to forestall a cold.
Varied Bath Products. The Body Shop; call 1-800-541-2535 for catalog. This British-based firm specializes in products made with natural ingredients such as herbal bath oils, massage oils, Body Buddy rubber mitt, exfoliating cactus brushes and mitts.

Herbal Products

Aloe Products. Aloe Flex Products, 1-800-231-0839. This Texas company grows its own aloe for topical use: tennis elbow, carpal tunnel syndrome, burns (including radiation burns).
Arnica Tablets. Health stores and drugstores carrying homeopathic products; Vitamin Shoppes, 1-800-223-1216 for catalog of homeopathic items. For body trauma, aches, pains, postsurgical problems, for use before dental surgery.
Calendula Ointment. Available at health stores or from Weleda; call 1-800-241-1030 for catalog. This healing salve is made from marigolds. Weleda also makes a variety of all-natural body care products from their own gardens, where they practice companion planting and other natural methods to eliminate pests. Products include chamomile extract, arnica massage oil, body lotions, baby care products and mouth products.
Castor Oil. Palma Christi Castor Oil. The Heritage Store, PO Box 44-U, Virginia Beach, VA 23458-0444. For effective healing compresses and packs.
Melisana. M.C.M. Klosterfrau, D 5000 Cologne 1, Germany. A remarkable German carminative (anti-gas) made from an ancient convent recipe. A few drops in a glass of water are used for gastric relief; can also be used topically for muscle soreness.
Olbas Massage Oil, Analgesic Oil, Ointment and Lotion. Available at health stores or call Penn Herb Co., Ltd. (Philadelphia, PA 19123-3098), 1-800-523-9771 for catalog.
Slippery Elm Lozenges. Available at health stores or write Henry Thayer Company, Concord, MA 01742. These have been comforting irritated throats for a century and a half.
Swedish Bitters. Available at health stores or write Nature Works, Inc., Agoura Hills, CA 91301. A herb tonic and restorative with 10 herbs plus aloe (a laxative when taken internally).
Tiger Balm. Health stores and drugstores. An Asian herbal analgesic ointment, available in white and red formulations; red is stronger but may stain clothes. Alternate with arnica ointment for muscle and other aches; a whiff of Tiger Balm may avert a sinus attack.
Zostrix. In pharmacy section of drugstores, but it's a nonprescription item. This topical analgesic's active ingredient is capsaicin (cayenne pepper); intended for relief of arthritis pain and neuralgias such as shingles (herpes zoster) or diabetic neuropathy. One of the few things besides

cool compresses, Aveeno and witch hazel compresses that can make life bearable during a shingles attack.

Allergy Aids

Negative Ion Generator. The Sharper Image, 1-800-344-5555.

Enviracaire Air Filtering System. Walnut Acres, Penns Creek, PA 17862, 1-800-283-9400. Said to remove tobacco smoke, bacteria, pollen dust, chemical fumes, pet hair, lint and other pollutants.

Humidifier. Hammacher Schlemmer; see listing under "Therapy Products Using Water," above.

Baby Products

All these are available from One Step Ahead, PO Box 517, Lake Bluff, IL 60044; for questions and catalog, 1-800-950-2120, weekdays 8 AM-11 PM Central Time; orders, 1-800-274-8440; fax (708) 615-2162.

Newborn Bathing. Baby Bather. This unique item is for that crucial time up to five months, when young parents are so tense. I remember taking the easy way and bathing my beloved in a small portable plastic "tub" in the kitchen sink. Now someone has invented a soft-as-air contour cushion that not only frees your hands but cradles the baby.

Six Months to Two Years. Baby Mooring Seat. No more slippery babies in the tub. Here is a collapsible, fitted seat that attaches to the tub, with easy straps for the baby. Your hands are miraculously free to make the child happy and comfortable.

Parent Knee Saver. Bathe'r Save'r. Older parents would have killed for this padded knee mat! Kneeling was never such fun.

Double Duty. Apron/Towel Hugger. Big enough for Mom or Dad, and when the bath ends you can hug the baby dry.

Index

ABOUT THE AUTHOR

DIAN DINCIN BUCHMAN is an expert in the field of natural health and natural medicine. She has a Ph.D. in Health Science, writes for *Health Quarterly,* and lectures extensively at colleges and universities. In the course of researching and writing this book, she interviewed over a hundred specialists—including internists, neurosurgeons, orthopedists, and professional athletic trainers—who use water therapy in treating their patients.

Dian Dincin Buchman comes from a long line of physicians who were pioneers in natural, nondrug medicine, both in Europe and America, and she has used water therapy with great success throughout her life to help maintain the good health of herself and her family. She lives in New York City.

Dr. Buchman is the author of *Herbal Medicine, The ABC's of Natural Beauty* and *The Complete Herbal Guide to Natural Health and Beauty*